Handbook of CTG Interpretation

T0177138

Handbook of CTG Interpretation

From Patterns to Physiology

Edited by
Edwin Chandraharan
St George's University Hospitals NHS Foundation Trust, London, and St George's University of London, UK

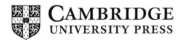
CAMBRIDGE
UNIVERSITY PRESS

CAMBRIDGE
UNIVERSITY PRESS

University Printing House, Cambridge CB2 8BS, United Kingdom

Cambridge University Press is part of the University of Cambridge.

It furthers the University's mission by disseminating knowledge in the pursuit of education, learning and research at the highest international levels of excellence.

www.cambridge.org
Information on this title: www.cambridge.org/9781107485501

© Cambridge University Press 2017

First published 2017
8th printing 2019

Printed in the United Kingdom by TJ International Ltd. Padstow Cornwall

A catalogue record for this publication is available from the British Library

Library of Congress Cataloging-in-Publication data
Names: Chandraharan, Edwin, editor.
Title: Handbook of CTG interpretation: from patterns to physiology / edited by Edwin Chandraharan.
Description: Cambridge, United Kingdom; New York:
Cambridge University Press, [2017] |
Includes bibliographical references and index.
Identifiers: LCCN 2016047896 | ISBN 9781107485501 (pbk.)
Subjects: | MESH: Cardiotocography | Fetal Hypoxia – prevention & control | Fetal Heart – physiology | Uterine Monitoring – methods
Classification: LCC RG618 | NLM WQ 209 | DDC 618.3261–dc23
LC record available at https://lccn.loc.gov/2016047896

ISBN 978-1-107-48550-1 Paperback

Dedicated to all babies who have sustained intrapartum hypoxic injuries and to all healthcare providers who are focussed on reflective practice

and

To my teachers who inspired me to develop an interest in human physiology and intrapartum care

Contents

Contributors

Anthony Addei, MB ChB, FRCA
Consultant Anaesthetist, St George's University Hospitals NHS Foundation Trust, UK

Anuji Amarasekara, MBBS, FRCA
Consultant Anaesthetist at the University Hospital of Coventry and Warwickshire, UK

Abigail Archer, BSc (Hons), RM
Specialist Midwife in Fetal Monitoring, St George's University Hospitals NHS Foundation Trust, London, UK

Sir Sabaratnam Arulkumaran PhD DSc FRCS FRCOG
Professor Emeritus of Obstetrics & Gynaecology
St George's University of London, UK

Amar Bhide, MD, FRCOG
Consultant, Fetal Medicine Unit, St George's University Hospitals NHS Foundation Trust, London, UK

Ana Piñas Carrillo, LMS, CCT Obs & Gyn (Spain), Dip FM (UK)
Consultant Obstetrician at St George's University Hospitals NHS Foundation Trust, London, UK

Edwin Chandraharan, MBBS, MS (Obs & Gyn), DFSRH, DCRM, FSLCOG, FRCOG
Lead Consultant, Labour Ward, St George's University Hospitals NHS Foundation Trust, and Honorary Senior Lecturer, St George's, University of London, UK. Visiting Professor, Tianjin Hospital for Obstetrics and Gynaecology, Tianjin Province, China

Francesco D'Antonio, MD
Clinical Fellow, Fetal Medicine Unit, St George's Hospital, London, UK

Madhusree Ghosh, MBBS, DNB (Obs & Gyn)
Clinical Fellow in Obstetrics and Gynaecology, St George's University Hospitals NHS Foundation Trust, London, UK

Anna Gracia-Perez-Bonfils, MD
Consultant Obstetrician
Sant Joan de Déu Hospital. BcnNatal. Barcelona, Spain

Dovilé Kalvinskaité, MD
Clinical Fellow (Obs & Gyn), St George's University Hospitals NHS Foundation Trust, London, UK

Sophie Eleanor Kay, MBBS, BSc (Hons)
Clinical Fellow, Women's Directorate, St George's University Hospitals NHS Foundation Trust, London, UK

Sabrina Kuah, MBBS, FRANZCOG, Diploma in Clinical Hypnosis
Director of Delivery Suite and Senior Consultant, Women's and Children's Hospital, Adelaide, South Australia

Sara Ledger, BSc (Hons)
Research and Development Manager, Baby Lifeline Training Ltd., Balsall Common, UK

Virginia Lowe, BA (Hons), BSc (Hons), RM
Specialist Midwife in Fetal Monitoring, St George's University Hospitals NHS Foundation Trust, London, UK

Geoff Matthews, BM, BS, FRCOG, FRANZCOG, RCR/RCOG, Diploma in Obstetric Ultrasound, Diploma in Clinical Hypnosis
Director of Obstetrics and Senior Consultant, Women's and Children's Hospital, Adelaide, South Australia

Charis Mills, MBBS, MSc
Clinical Fellow in Obstetrics and Gynaecology, Women's Directorate, St George's University Hospitals NHS Foundation Trust, London, UK

Jessica Moore, MBBS, MRCOG
Consultant Obstetrician and Lead for Obstetric Risk Management, St George's University Hospitals NHS Foundation Trust, London, UK

Sadia Muhammad, MBBS, MRCOG
Senior Lecturer and Head of Department of Obstetrics and Gynaecology, Faculty of MedicineUniversity of JaffnaSri Lanka

K. Muhunthan, MBBS, MS (Obs & Gyn), MRCOG
Senior Lecturer, Consultant and Head Department of Obstetrics and Gynaecology, Faculty of Medicine, University of Jaffna, Sri Lanka

Leonie Penna, FRCOG
Consultant, Obstetrician Department of Women's Health, King's College Hospital, London, UK

Nirmala Chandrasekaran, MRCOG
Senior Registrar at the Department of Women's Health, King's College Hospital, London, UK

Justin Richards, MBBS, MD, MRCP
Consultant Neonatologist, St George's University Hospitals NHS Foundation Trust, London, UK

Abigail Spring, MBChB (Hons)
Clinical Fellow in Obstetrics and Gynaecology, St George's University Hospitals NHS Foundation Trust, London, UK

Harriet Stevenson, MBBS, iBsc
Clinical Fellow, St George's University Hospitals NHS Foundation Trust, London, UK

Mary Catherine Tolcher, MD
Department of Obstetrics and Gynecology, Mayo Clinic, Rochester, MN, USA

Rosemary Townsend, MBChB, MRCOG
Specialist Trainee, St George's University Hospitals NHS Foundation Trust, London, UK

Kyle D. Traynor, MD
Department of Obstetrics and Gynecology, Mayo Clinic, Rochester, MN, USA

Austin Ugwumadu, PhD, FRCOG
Consultant and Senior Lecturer in Obstetrics and Gynaecology, St George's University of London, UK

Ayona Wijemanne, BMedSci, BMBS, MRCOG, DCRM
Clinical Fellow in Obstetrics and Gynaecology, St George's University Hospitals NHS Foundation Trust, London, UK

Preface

Why do we need a textbook on physiology-based cardiotocograph (CTG) interpretation? In order to answer this question, one needs to look at the recent '10 Years of Maternity Claims' report published by the NHS Litigation Authority (NHSLA) in 2013, which highlighted the fact that even 40 years after CTG was introduced into clinical practice, CTG misinterpretation continues to contribute to significant number of clinical negligence claims involving cerebral palsy and perinatal deaths.

Very unfortunately, CTG technology was introduced into clinical practice in 1968 without any randomized controlled trials to confirm its effectiveness in reducing perinatal morbidity and mortality. Lack of deep understanding of the features observed on the CTG trace led to early CTG 'experts' reacting to various 'concerning' features without understanding the basic pathophysiological mechanisms behind these patterns. Fetal stress response was mistaken as fetal 'distress', leading to unnecessary intrapartum interventions such as operative vaginal deliveries and emergency caesarean sections. Conversely, the lack of deeper understanding of CTG trace features (failure to recognize features suggestive of fetal decompensation) resulted in adverse perinatal outcomes, including hypoxic ischaemic encephalopathy and its long-term sequelae such as cerebral palsy.

One of the main reasons for substandard care associated with CTG interpretation was because CTG was introduced into clinical practice in 1960s without robust guidelines as to how to use this technology. The first clinical guidelines were published by the American College of Obstetricians and Gynaecologists (ACOG) in 1979, although there were a few 'expert opinions' in existence between 1968 and 1979. In early 1980s, there were more than 20 CTG classification systems employed around the world, leading to significant confusion among obstetricians and midwives about how to use this technology effectively. This compelled the International Federation of Gynaecology and Obstetrics (FIGO) to produce the first unified clinical guidelines on CTG interpretation in 1987 (19 years after the introduction of CTG into clinical practice!). In the United Kingdom, the first ever guidelines on CTG interpretation were published by the Royal College of Obstetricians and Gynaecologists (RCOG) only in 2001, after the fourth 'Confidential Enquiries into Stillbirths and Deaths in Infancy' (CESDI) report in 1997. This report highlighted that the lack of knowledge with CTG interpretation was a key contributory factor in intrapartum-related stillbirths.

Unfortunately, all these guidelines that have been published so far were highly dependent on 'pattern recognition' to classify CTG traces. They have relied on morphological identification of ongoing decelerations, which were classified initially as 'Type 1' and 'Type 2' and subsequently as 'early, variable and late' decelerations, with the variable decelerations further classified into typical (uncomplicated) and atypical (complicated) decelerations.

Not only do these decelerations not occur in isolation during labour, they are subjected to significant inter- and intra-observer variability, leading to misclassification. Studies have shown that even experts providing medico-legal evidence to courts who rely on 'pattern recognition' for CTG interpretation change their opinions when the neonatal outcome is known and completely revise their CTG classification based on the neonatal outcomes. This illustrates the confusion with regard to CTG interpretation even among experts.

The CESDI report in the United Kingdom highlighted the fact that out of 873 intrapartum-related deaths, 50% had 'grade 3' substandard care. This means that 50% of intrapartum deaths were potentially avoidable. Factors that contributed to substandard care included lack of knowledge to interpret CTG traces, failure to incorporate clinical picture (meconium, temperature, intrapartum bleeding), delay in interventions and communication and common sense issues. The Chief Medical Officer's report in 2006 on 'Intrapartum-Related Deaths: 500 Missed Opportunities' continued to highlight substandard care, including CTG misinterpretation, as a contributory factor. NHSLA published the '100 Stillbirth Claims' report in 2009, which indicated that out of 100 successful stillbirth claims, 34% were directly due to CTG misinterpretation involving both obstetricians and midwives. The most recent NHSLA's '10 Years of Maternity Claims' report has also highlighted CTG misinterpretation as a cornerstone of medical malpractice in maternity services leading to stillbirths, hypoxic ischaemic encephalopathy (HIE) and subsequent long-term sequelae such as cerebral palsy.

CTG misinterpretation not only has significant financial implications for any healthcare system because a single case of cerebral palsy may cost approximately £10 million; it also has an immeasurable adverse impact on families. A child with cerebral palsy requires round-the-clock intensive care, in addition to regular occupational therapy, speech and language therapy, almost on a weekly basis. Therefore, parents often have to lose their jobs to become full-time caregiverrs to look after their children. In addition, intrapartum stillbirth or an early neonatal death can also cause enormous emotional trauma, which may even affect subsequent pregnancies. Moreover, one should not forget the impact of CTG misinterpretation leading to poor outcomes on staff (midwives, obstetricians, anaesthetists and neonatologists). Some leave their chosen profession due to this negative psychological impact. Therefore, CTG misinterpretation does not only cause medico-legal implications leading to financial loss but also has a significant impact on individuals, families and, largely, the society.

Therefore, in my opinion, time has come for a paradigm shift in CTG interpretation from that based on traditional 'pattern recognition', which has led to significant inter- and intra-observer variation and resultant increase in operative interventions during labour without any significant reductions in the rates of cerebral palsy or perinatal deaths, to one based on fetal physiology. The latter is aimed at understanding the basic pathophysiology behind features observed on the CTG trace so as to institute a timely and appropriate action when there is evidence of fetal decompensation. Conversely, it would help to avoid an unnecessary intrapartum operative intervention when there is evidence of fetal compensation to ongoing mechanical or hypoxic stress on the CTG trace. Based on animal and human studies, it is very clear that a fetus when exposed to an evolving intrapartum hypoxia would display certain definitive and predictable features on the CTG trace, which reflect attempts at physiological compensation, similar to adults. Although the degree of response may vary depending on the intensity and duration of the hypoxic insult as well as the individual reserve of the given fetus, the fetal compensatory response to ongoing intrapartum hypoxia, which leads ultimately to decompensation, is fairly predictable.

It is important to realize that fetuses are not exposed to atmospheric oxygen and, therefore, are unable to increase the oxygenation of their myocardium by increasing the rate and depth of respiration. Therefore, in order to maintain a positive energy balance within the myocardium, a fetus needs to decrease its heart rate so as to decrease the workload of the myocardium in order to conserve energy. Therefore, one should not panic when observing decelerations on the CTG trace and should not merely classify them based on morphology into early, typical variable, atypical variable and late decelerations. Midwives and obstetricians caring for babies in labour need to consider decelerations as baro- and/or chemoreceptor responses to ongoing hypoxic or mechanical stresses. They should then attempt to determine the response of the fetus to ongoing hypoxic or mechanical stress by observing the features on the CTG trace in between the decelerations (i.e. stability of the baseline heart rate and normal variability) so as to intervene when a fetus shows evidence of decompensation. An intervention does not always indicate an immediate delivery using a vacuum or forceps or an emergency caesarean section. In contrast, the intervention should be always aimed at improving intrauterine environment wherever possible, even if delivery subsequently becomes necessary. Except in cases of acute intrapartum accidents (abruption, cord prolapse, scar rupture), when an immediate delivery is warranted, a fetus would display a definitive and predictable compensatory response to ongoing evolving hypoxic stress. Therefore, recognition of fetal compensation from decompensation is essential to manage labour.

The introductory chapters deal with normal fetal physiology and placentation as well as the technical aspects of the CTG machine. This is followed by use of CTG in various clinical situations and the pearls and pitfalls associated with CTG interpretation. Every attempt has been made to explain the fetal pathophysiological changes behind various features observed on the CTG trace and, where applicable, a 'CTG Exercise' is included after each chapter to test reader's knowledge. CTG changes in nonhypoxic brain injury aims to illustrate some of the rare conditions that one may encounter in clinical practice. Considering the fact that safe intrapartum care involves a joint, multidisciplinary effort, midwives, obstetricians, anaesthetists and neonatologists have contributed chapters on relevant areas, including intermittent auscultation, role of anaesthetists during an event of CTG changes, as well as neonatal resuscitation.

I would like to thank all the contributors for their hard work and sacrifice. They have ensured that chapters are based on current scientific evidence as well as on fetal pathophysiology. I am deeply indebted to my mentor Professor Sir Arulkumaran who inspired me to develop an interest in intrapartum fetal monitoring. Special thanks to my colleagues Mr Ugwumadu, Ms Leonie Penna, Ms Virginia Whelehan and Ms Abigail Archer, who are co-members of the faculty of St George's intrapartum fetal monitoring courses. I would like to thank Ms Sara Ledger from Baby Lifeline, a charity which conducts CTG masterclasses for midwives and obstetricians in several regions in the United Kingdom for her contribution on delegate feedback on physiology-based CTG interpretation. My special appreciation goes to all my co-authors, who were or are my trainees and have been interpreting CTG traces based on fetal physiology and are extremely motivated to improve intrapartum outcomes. They are our leaders of tomorrow, and I have no doubt whatsoever that they will be pivotal in changing the way the CTG has been interpreted based on pattern recognition over the last 40 years and that they would ensure a culture change to move towards a physiology-based CTG interpretation to improve outcomes for women and babies.

I sincerely hope that this book will help start our journey towards a physiology-based CTG interpretation. We owe this to women and babies who place their trust in us to care for them during labour.

Acknowledgements

I would like to thank all the contributing authors for their generosity with their time, dissemination of their knowledge and expertise. As the labour ward lead, my sincere appreciation goes to the multidisciplinary team at St George's University Hospitals NHS Trust, London, for their continued support and assistance.

I am very grateful to Mr Nick Dunton, Ms Kirsten Bot and their team at the Cambridge University Press for their invaluable support and assistance as well as their professionalism.

I am deeply indebted to my wife Anomi and my children Ashane and Avindri not only for their unconditional support, always, but also for their patience, tolerance and understanding.

Last but not least, my thanks to all the babies who have taught me the importance of incorporating fetal physiology during labour while interpreting CTG traces over the last 20 years.

Glossary

Augmentation of labour: The process of artificially stimulating the uterus to increase the frequency, duration and intensity of uterine contractions after the onset of spontaneous labour. It is indicated when labour is progressing slowly or not progressing at all so as to avoid the complications secondary to prolonged labour.

Bradycardia: A baseline fetal heart rate <110 bpm for at least 10 minutes.

Cardiotocography – CTG: A graphic record of the fetal heart rate and uterine contractions through an ultrasound device placed on the maternal abdomen or through a fetal scalp electrode. The 'toco', registers the uterine contractions through a second transducer placed on the uterine fundus.

Induction of labour – IOL: The process of artificially initiating the onset of labour so as to optimize maternal and/or fetal outcome by avoiding continuation of pregnancy.

Intermittent auscultation: A method of intrapartum surveillance where the fetal heart rate is heard for short periods of time at prespecified intervals.

Intrapartum bleeding: Any bleeding from the genital tract that is heavier than the usually expected blood-stained mucus discharge during labour.

Intrapartum reoxygenation ratio – IRR: The ratio between cumulative uterine relaxation and uterine contraction times over 30 minutes indicates the total duration of time available for reoxygenation of placental venous sinuses, immediately after a uterine contraction during a 30-minute period. IRR >1 (i.e. relaxation time is more than the time spent during a contraction) is unlikely to lead to fetal hypoxia and acidosis.

Intrauterine resuscitation: Any intervention undertaken during labour with the aim/intention to improve oxygen delivery to the fetus by improving the intrauterine environment.

Meconium: Fetal bowel content that is passed into the amniotic fluid in about 10 percent of term labours. The term meconium-stained amniotic fluid is used to describe this situation. The terms "light" meconium staining and "heavy" meconium staining are recommended with the former representing a situation that is most likely physiological with a large volume of amniotic fluid indicating a lower risk of placental insufficiency or prolonged ruptured membranes, and the latter indicating a situation in which the fetus may have oligohydramnios due to placental insufficiency, prolonged prelabour rupture of membranes or a long labour and is thus more likely to be associated with hypoxia or infection.

MHR: Maternal heart rate. Erroneous recording of MHR on cardiotocography may be misinterpreted as the fetal heart rate (FHR)

Operative vaginal delivery (with vacuum or forceps)/cesarean delivery: These are options for management of "pathological" (or a 'category 3') cardiotocography observed during second stage of labour.

Peripheral tests of fetal well-being: These are aimed at testing a sample of blood taken from fetal scalp to determine fetal acidosis (fetal scalp pH or scalp lactate) or to assess oxygenation saturation from fetal skin (fetal pulse oximetry).

Preterm: All fetuses between 24 weeks (considered as the limit of viability) and 37 completed weeks (the 259th day).

Prolonged deceleration: Fall from baseline fetal heart rate of >15 beats per minute lasting longer than 3 minutes.

Sinusoidal pattern: A regular oscillation of baseline variability in a smooth undulating pattern lasting at least 10 minutes with a frequency of 3–5 cycles per minute and an amplitude of 5 to 15 bpm above and below the baseline.

STAN: A system of intrapartum monitoring that records changes in fetal ECG during labour. It analyses the 'ST segment' and the 'T-wave' of the fetal ECG complex.

Uterine scar: Any interruption in the integrity of the myometrium and its subsequent replacement by scar tissue before pregnancy. Although a previous caesarean section is the most common cause of uterine scarring, a previous myomectomy, uterine perforation/rupture, resection of cornual ectopic pregnancy and any other procedure that involves an interruption of the myometrium with subsequent replacement by scar tissue may weaken the uterine wall, predisposing to uterine scar dehiscence or rupture.

Zig-zag (saltatory) autonomic instability pattern: Fetal heart amplitude changes of >25 bpm with an oscillatory frequency of >6 per minute for a minimum duration of 1 minute.

'An Eye Opener': Perils of CTG Misinterpretation

Lessons from Confidential Enquiries and Medico-legal Cases

Edwin Chandraharan

Introduction

Since its introduction into clinical practice in late 1960s, cardiotocograph (CTG) interpretation was predominantly based on 'pattern recognition' by determining various features observed on the CTG trace (e.g. baseline fetal heart rate [FHR], baseline variability, presence of accelerations and decelerations). One of the main reasons for this approach was due to the fact that the CTG was first introduced to clinical practice without any robust randomized controlled clinical trials to confirm its efficacy. Very unfortunately, robust guidelines on how to use this new technology were not published at the time of introduction of CTG into clinical practice. This unfortunate situation resulted in obstetricians in late 1960s and early 1970s reacting to various patterns observed on the CTG trace without understanding the pathophysiological mechanisms behind these observed features. The first recognized guidelines on CTG interpretation were published by the American College of Obstetricians and Gynaecologists (ACOG) in 1979, and subsequent international guidelines on CTG interpretation were published by the International Federation of Gynecology and Obstetrics (FIGO) in 1987 as there were more than 20 international guidelines at this time on how to interpret the CTG trace. Lack of understanding of pathophysiology of intrapartum hypoxia as well as randomized controlled trials on CTG resulted in obstetricians merely exerting a panic reaction to observed decelerations, which were initially termed 'type 1' and 'type 2' decelerations, and this resulted in increased operative interventions (emergency caesarean sections, operative vaginal births) without any significant reduction in cerebral palsy and perinatal deaths.

Effects of CTG Misinterpretation

In 1971, Beard et al. reported that even when significant abnormalities (e.g. late decelerations and complicated baseline bradycardia) were noted on the CTG trace, more than 60 per cent of fetuses had a normal umbilical cord pH (>7.25). Therefore, CTG interpretation purely based on 'pattern recognition' resulted in unnecessary caesarean sections. As the false-positive rate of CTG was 60 per cent, out of 100 caesarean sections performed, 60 were potentially unnecessary. However, due to a paucity of knowledge with regard to

Handbook of CTG Interpretation: From Patterns to Physiology, ed. Edwin Chandraharan. Published by Cambridge University Press. © Cambridge University Press 2017.

fetal acid–base balance during labour in the late 1960s and 1970s, it was thought, based on personal opinions of a few senior obstetricians, that if the fetal pH was 7.25 or less, 'it is considered possible that the fetus was asphyxiated'. Subsequent large observational studies have refuted this erroneous assumption, and it is now well known that the cord arterial pH of less than 7.0 (and not 7.25) is associated with poor perinatal outcomes. Therefore, if a cut-off of 7.0 was used instead of 7.25 by Beard et al. in 1971, it was very likely that the false-positive rate of CTG would have been over 90 per cent. This implies that, if pattern recognition is used for CTG interpretation without understanding the fetal physiology, 90 out of 100 emergency caesarean sections performed for suspected fetal compromise would be entirely avoidable.

CTG misinterpretation has an adverse impact on the fetuses, their families as well as the society. In 1997, the fourth 'Confidential Enquiries into Stillbirths and Deaths in Infancy' (CESDI) reported that more than 50 per cent of intrapartum-related stillbirths were due to 'grade 3' substandard care, and, therefore, approximately 400 out of 873 stillbirths were potentially avoidable by an alternative management. Lack of knowledge in the interpretation of CTG traces, failure to incorporate the entire clinical picture (meconium, maternal temperature, chorioamnionitis, etc.), delay in intervention even after recognizing an abnormality on the CTG, as well as communication and common sense issues were the key identified areas in cases with substandard care.

The Chief Medical Officer's report in the United Kingdom in 2006 titled 'Intrapartum-Related Deaths: 500 Missed Opportunities' highlighted similar issues relating to substandard care even 10 years after the CESDI report in 1997. This was followed by the National Health Service Litigation Authority's (NHSLA) report on '100 Stillbirth Claims' in 2009, which highlighted the fact that 34 per cent of stillbirth claims involved CTG misinterpretation.

In addition to poor perinatal outcomes and long-term neurological sequelae, CTG misinterpretation is also associated with significant medico-legal costs. Vincent and Ennis reported issues relating to poor record-keeping and storage of CTG traces as contributory factors.

The more recent NHSLA's '10 Years of Maternity Claims' report highlighted the medico-legal implications of CTG misinterpretation, which contributed not only to claims arising from cerebral palsy and stillbirths but also to complications arising out of emergency caesarean sections. Failure to recognize an abnormal CTG, failure to incorporate clinical picture, failure in communication and injudicious use of oxytocin infusion were highlighted as key contributory factors to medico-legal claims. The overall cost of medico-legal claims was over three billion pounds.

The issues relating to CTG misinterpretation are not unique to the United Kingdom. Recent publications from Norway have suggested that substandard care is common in birth asphyxia cases, and *human error* is the most common contributory factor. Similar publications from Sweden have highlighted that injudicious use of oxytocin in labour was associated with approximately 70 per cent of all medico-legal claims.

The author's own medico-legal practice, analysis of the CTG trace as well as management of labour suggested that approximately 70 per cent of all cases of cerebral palsy and perinatal mortality were potentially avoidable by an alternative management. In addition, poor CTG interpretation may lead to an unnecessary intrapartum operative intervention such as fetal scalp blood sampling (FBS), operative vaginal delivery as well as an emergency caesarean section, all of which are associated with potentially serious maternal and fetal complications.

In June 2016, the Royal College of Obstetricians and Gynaecologists published 'Each Baby Counts: key messages from 2015'. There were 921 *reported* cases in 2015 comprising of

119 intrapartum deaths, 147 early neonatal deaths and 655 babies with severe brain injury in the UK.

CTG Interpretation: What Is the Problem?

One of the main drawbacks of CTG is that it was introduced into clinical practice without any robust randomized controlled trials. Due to the lack of knowledge of fetal physiology in the 1960s when the CTG technology was developing, obstetricians who worked with the technology very unfortunately reacted to various patterns that were observed on the CTG trace since no proper guidelines as to how to use the technology were made available to the practitioners! Although several attempts were made by obstetricians working with the technology to produce an acceptable methodology of CTG classification, the first robust guidelines were only produced in 1979 by ACOG. This was followed by the production of CTG guidelines by FIGO in 1987 to have a consensus in view of several different guidelines in use around the world, each adopting different features and classification systems at that time.

The initial panic attacks caused by the 'decelerations' observed on the CTG trace resulted in an exponential increase in operative vaginal births as well as emergency caesarean sections without any significant reductions in cerebral palsy or perinatal deaths. Obstetricians in 1960s and early 1970s were indeed very surprised to observe babies being born in a very good condition with vigorous crying when obstetricians had thought that they were experiencing 'asphyxia' based on the observed decelerations on the CTG trace. Professor Richard Beard's study in 1971 caused further confusion among obstetricians when he demonstrated that even when severe abnormalities were noted on the CTG trace, approximately 60 per cent of neonates were born with a normal acid–base balance (arterial umbilical cord pH >7.25).

This led to some obstetricians introducing a test called FBS, which was developed by Erich Saling in Germany in 1962 as an alternative to a Pinard's stethoscope. FBS was never validated as an additional or adjunctive test to the CTG prior to its introduction into clinical practice. It was merely introduced as a 'knee-jerk reaction' in response to Beard's publication to reduce the false-positive rate of CTG so as to avoid unnecessary caesarean sections.

Such decelerations that were reflex responses of a fetus to a hypoxic or mechanical stress in labour in order to protect the myocardium as well as changes secondary to increased systemic blood pressure during umbilical cord compression were thought to be 'pathological'. This erroneous assumption without a deeper understanding of fetal physiology resulted in such classifications as 'type 1' and 'type 2' decelerations, leading to further panic attacks among obstetricians and an increase in unnecessary intrapartum operative interventions. Conversely, a failure to appreciate the significance of abnormalities observed on the CTG trace resulted in intrapartum stillbirths, hypoxic-ischaemic encephalopathy (HIE) and its long-term sequelae such as cerebral palsy and learning difficulties, as well as early neonatal deaths.

The vast majority of current guidelines on CTG interpretation are purely based on 'pattern recognition', and some of these guidelines force obstetricians to perform an FBS for a 'pathological' CTG despite current evidence from the *Cochrane Database of Systematic Reviews* confirming that FBS, unlike what was believed by some senior obstetricians in the past, neither reduces operative interventions nor improves long-term perinatal outcomes. In contrast, FBS may be associated with potentially serious fetal complications (including severe haemorrhage, sepsis and leakage of cerebrospinal fluid) and may in fact delay delivery by up to 18 minutes.

In addition, several publications have highlighted that the interpretation of CTG is fraught with both inter- and intra-observer variations. Therefore, merely classifying CTG traces based on pattern recognition would lead not only to erroneous interpretations but also to unnecessary intrapartum operative interventions as well as delays in intervention.

Therefore, there is an urgent need to go back to basic fetal physiology to understand the pathophysiology behind the features observed on the CTG trace so as to treat the fetus rather than merely classifying the CTG trace into normal, suspicious or pathological. There is an urgent need, first, to appreciate that intrapartum fetal monitoring is all about ensuring that the fetus is not exposed to any significant hypoxic stress, and, second, to differentiate between a fetus that is able to and one that is unable to mount a successful compensatory response to ongoing stress or has exhausted all the means of compensation and hence has begun the process of decompensation. Therefore, features observed on the CTG traces should be used to understand fetal pathophysiology in order to avoid inappropriate interventions.

Midwives and obstetricians caring for women must avoid unnecessary operative interventions during labour while ensuring optimum perinatal outcome by developing a deeper understanding of fetal physiology.

Further Reading

1. Beard RW, Filshie GM, Knight CA, Roberts GM. The significance of the changes in the continuous fetal heart rate in the first stage of labour. *J Obstet Gynaecol Br Commonw*. 1971; 78: 865–881.

2. Chauhan SP, Klauser CK, Woodring TC, Sanderson M, Magann EF, Morrison JC. Intrapartum nonreassuring fetal heart rate tracing and prediction of adverse outcomes: interobserver variability. *Am J ObstetGynecol*. 2008; 199: 623.e1–623.e5.

3. NHSLA. Study of stillbirth claims. 2009. www.nhsla.com/safety/Documents/ NHS%20Litigation%20Authority%20 Study%20of%20Stillbirth%20Claims.pdf

4. NHSLA. Ten years of maternity claims: An analysis of NHS litigation authority data. 2012. www.nhsla.com/safety/Documents/ Ten%20Years%20of%20Maternity%20 Claims%20-%20An%20Analysis%20 of%20the%20NHS%20LA%20Data%20- %20October%202012.pdf

5. Chandraharan E. Fetal compromise: diagnosis and management. In: *Obstetric and Intrapartum Emergencies: A Practical Guide to Management*. Cambridge University Press, 2012.

6. Chandraharan E, Lowe V, Penna L, Ugwumadu A, Arulkumaran S. Does 'process based' training in fetal monitoring improve knowledge of Cardiotocograph (CTG) among midwives and obstetricians? In: *Book of Abstracts*. Ninth RCOG International Scientific Meeting, Athens, 2011. www.rcog.org.uk/events/rcog- congresses/athens-2011

7. Ayres-de-Campos D, Arteiro D, Costa-Santos C, Bernardes J. Knowledge of adverse neonatal outcome alters clinicians' interpretation of the intrapartum cardiotocograph. *BJOG*. 2011; 118(8): 978–984.

8. Chandraharan E. Fetal scalp blood sampling during labour: is it a useful diagnostic test or a historical test that no longer has a place in modern clinical obstetrics? *BJOG*. 2014; 121(9): 1056–1060.

9. Department of Health, UK. On the state of public health: annual report of the Chief Medical Officer 2006. Chapter 6. Intrapartum-Related Deaths: 500 Missed Opportunities. webarchive. nationalarchives.gov.uk/20130107105354/ http://www.dh.gov.uk/prod_consum_ dh/groups/dh_digitalassets/@dh/@en/ documents/digitalasset/dh_076853.pdf

10. CESDI. Fourth Annual Report: Concentrating on Intrapartum Deaths 1994-95. London. Maternal and Child Health Research Consortium, 1997.

11. Ennis M, Vincent CA. Obstetric accidents: a review of 64 cases. *BMJ*. 1990; 300(6736): 1365–1367.

12. Berglund S, Grunewald C, Pettersson H, Cnattingius S. Severe asphyxia due to delivery-related malpractice in Sweden 1990–2005. *BJOG*. 2008; 115(3): 316–323.

13. Andreasen S, Backe B, Øian P. Claims for compensation after alleged birth asphyxia: a nationwide study covering 15 years. *Acta Obstet Gynecol Scand*. 2014; 93(2): 152–158.

14. Royal College of Obstetricans and Gynaecologists. Each baby Counts: key messages from 2015. London: RCOG2016.

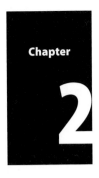

Chapter

2

Fetal Oxygenation

Anna Gracia-Perez-Bonfils and Edwin Chandraharan

Introduction

Fetuses, unlike adults, are not exposed to atmospheric oxygen. When confronted with hypoxia, adults can increase their rate and depth of respiration to enhance the intake of oxygen so as to maintain positive energy balance and protect their myocardium.

In contrast, a fetus when exposed to hypoxia cannot increase its oxygen supply, and therefore, it will decrease its heart rate in order to reduce the myocardial workload to maintain a positive energy balance. This reflex response to decrease the heart rate to protect the myocardium against hypoxic or mechanical stress is heard as a deceleration during fetal heart rate (FHR) monitoring.

Placentation: Impact on Fetal Oxygenation

From 12 days of life until full-term, the embryo and the fetus obtain their nutrition and oxygenation from maternal circulation to survive and grow. Therefore, it is mandatory for the well-being of an embryo and a fetus to have optimum utero-placental circulation as well as adequate placental reserve. This process of establishing an effective utero-placental circulation is complex and requires a synergy between the trophoblasts of the embryo and the endometrium (decidua and spiral arterioles) of the mother.

Normal Placentation

Fertilization occurs in the fallopian tube, and the fertilized ovum enters the uterine cavity around the third day as a morula (12–16 blastomeres). The inner cells of the morula differentiate into an inner cell mass that will form the tissues of the embryo. In contrast, the surrounding cells differentiate into the outer cell mass that will give rise to the trophoblast, which will subsequently form the placenta.

The accumulation of fluid occurs rapidly forming a fluid-filled cavity within the morula (blastocele) and thereby creating the blastocyst. During this time, the early embryo receives its nutrition and eliminates waste products by a simple process of diffusion through the zona pellucida. About the sixth day, the cells from the trophoblast begin to penetrate between the endometrial cells of the uterus.

The process of implantation is usually completed by the tenth or eleventh postovulatory day. By that time, the original trophoblast surrounding the embryo has undergone differentiation

Handbook of CTG Interpretation: From Patterns to Physiology, ed. Edwin Chandraharan. Published by Cambridge University Press. © Cambridge University Press 2017.

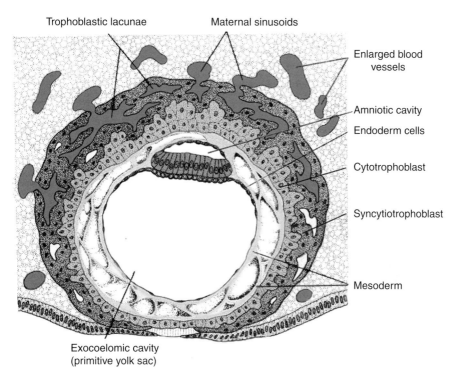

Trophoblastic lacunae   Maternal sinusoids

Enlarged blood
vessels

Amniotic cavity

Endoderm cells

Cytotrophoblast

Syncytiotrophoblast

Mesoderm

Exocoelomic cavity
(primitive yolk sac)

Figure 2.1 Formation of primitive utero-placental circulation by erosion of maternal blood vessels by syncytiotrophoblast.

into two layers: the inner cytotrophoblast and the outer syncytiotrophoblast, which will invade the endometrium and subsequently form the placenta.

The growth of the embryo and the disappearance of the zona pellucida induce a need for a new and more efficient method of exchange of nutrients. This need is fulfilled by the utero-placental circulation that allows a close contact to exchange gases and metabolites by diffusion between maternal and fetal blood. The formation of 'lacunae' within the syncytio-trophoblast aids in the development of an efficient utero-placental circulation.

The uterus at the time of implantation is in the secretory phase, and secondary to the rise in concentration of progesterone, the stroma cells of the endometrium accumulate glycogen and get enlarged. On day 12, the syncytiotrophoblast secretes enzymes that erode the endometrium and hormones that help to sustain ongoing pregnancy (B-hCG). Enzymatic corrosion of uterine glands liberates their content for nourishment of the embryo, together with the glycogen provided by the stromal cells. Maternal vessels at the implantation site (branches of spiral arteries and endometrial veins) dilate and form maternal sinusoids. The erosion of sinusoids by the syncytiotrophoblast results in maternal blood bathing the lacunar network allowing the exchange of gases and nutrients (Figure 2.1). Thus, a primitive utero-placental circulation begins by the end of the second week with the anastomosis between trophoblastic lacunae and maternal capillaries.

These cellular changes, together with an increase in endometrial vascularization, are known as decidual reaction. It commences at the implantation site and spreads throughout

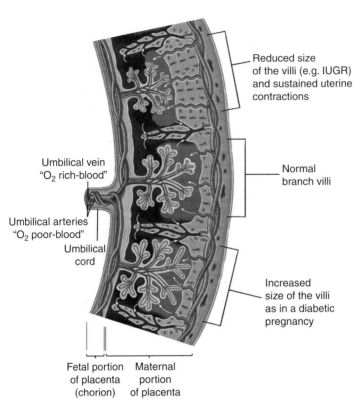

Reduced size
of the villi (e.g. IUGR)
and sustained uterine
contractions

Umbilical vein
"O$_2$ rich-blood"

Umbilical arteries
"O$_2$ poor-blood"

Umbilical
cord

Normal
branch villi

Increased
size of the villi
as in a diabetic
pregnancy

Fetal portion   Maternal
of placenta   portion
(chorion)   of placenta

Figure 2.2 Maternal spiral arteries and their branches as well as the intervillous space formed by the intercommunicating lacunae within the trophoblast. The terminal branches of spiral arterioles feed oxygenated blood while the tributaries of the endometrial veins drain deoxygenated blood and metabolic waste products.

the entire endometrium within a few days, and this newly formed layer is called the *decidua*. As the trophoblast continues to invade more and more sinusoids, maternal blood begins to flow through the trophoblastic system.

The cytotrophoblast meanwhile proliferates and forms protrusions penetrating into the syncytiotrophoblast all around the blastocyst. These extensions are known as primary villi. On day 16, after being invaded by the chorionic mesoderm, secondary villi are formed. This is followed by the development of blood vessels within the chorionic mesoderm leading to the formation of tertiary villi on day 21. Secondary and tertiary villi are often termed as chorionic villi, and hypoxia or lower tissue oxygen content in the decidua is critical for normal trophoblast invasion and formation of these villi.

The embryonic circulation is anatomically separated from the maternal circulation by the endothelium of the villus capillaries, the connective tissue in the core of the villus, a layer of cytotrophoblast and a layer of syncytiotrophoblast.

By the end of fourth week, tertiary stem villi surround the entire chorion and establish contact with the extraembryonic circulatory system, connecting the placenta and the embryo (Figure 2.2). This ensures that nutrients and oxygen are supplied to the fetus and metabolic waste products are removed when the fetal heart begins to start beating.

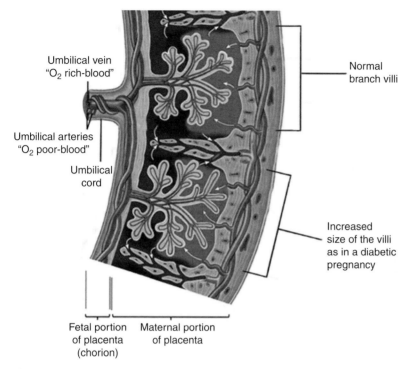

Umbilical vein
"O_2 rich-blood"

Normal
branch villi

Umbilical arteries
"O_2 poor-blood"

Umbilical
cord

Increased
size of the villi
as in a diabetic
pregnancy

Fetal portion   Maternal portion
of placenta   of placenta
(chorion)

Figure 2.3 Impaired placental circulation in a diabetic pregnancy secondary to hyperplacentosis and resultant reduction in the utero-placental pool.

Impact of Placental Reserve on Fetal Growth and Well-being

If the placental reserve is low (utero-placental sinuses are smaller) during the antenatal period, the fetus might have restricted his/her growth to supply oxygenated blood to the vital organs. During labour, the onset of uterine contractions might lead to a rapid development of hypoxia and acidosis due to the compression of branches of the uterine artery by the contracting myometrial fibres. Similarly, an injudicious use of oxytocin may increase the frequency, duration and strength of uterine contractions and thereby reduce the perfusion of utero-placental sinuses leading to the development of hypoxia and metabolic acidosis. Similarly in diabetic pregnancies, hyper-placentosis may reduce the amount of placental pools available for gaseous exchange (Figure 3.3) leading to a rapid development of hypoxia and acidosis.

Fetal Adaptation to Hypoxic Intrauterine Environment

The fetus lives in a relatively hypoxic intrauterine environment with an arterial oxygen saturation of 70 per cent prior to the onset of labour. During labour, intermittent uterine contractions may further reduce fetal oxygen saturation down to 30 per cent. Unlike adults, a fetus has 18–22 g of fetal haemoglobin, which helps to increase the oxygen-carrying capacity of fetal blood. In addition, unlike adult haemoglobin (HbA), fetal haemoglobin (HbF) has increased affinity for oxygen. This results in the binding of oxygen molecules at higher partial pressures of oxygen and the releasing of oxygen rapidly at very low oxygen tensions.

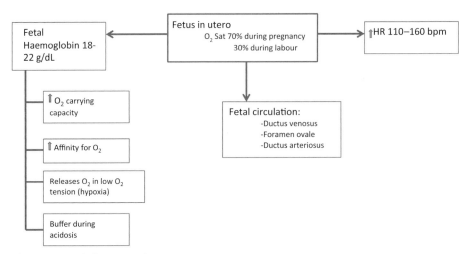

Figure 2.4 Fetal adaptation to hypoxia.

This enables the fetus to maintain adequate oxygenation of the central organs even when it is not exposed to external environment. Moreover, an increased level of fetal haemoglobin acts as an effective buffering system in the presence of metabolic acidosis to help avoid fetal neurological damage (Figure 2.4).

The fetal circulatory system consists of ductus venosus and foramen ovale, both of which preferentially shunt oxygenated blood from the umbilical vein to the heart and the brain (vital organs). In addition, ductus arteriosus diverts the blood from the pulmonary artery to the descending aorta by passing nonfunctional lungs. This vascular arrangement enables the fetus to supply the central organs with relatively well-oxygenated blood as compared to the peripheral tissues. In order to rapidly distribute the blood to vital organs, unlike in adults, fetal myocardium beats at a higher rate (110–160 bpm).

Abnormal Placentation

A failure of trophoblast invasion into the uterine endometrium would result in inadequate formation of placental lacunae. This would lead to a reduction in the size of pools of oxygenated blood within the uterine venous sinuses. Therefore, there may be intrauterine growth restriction (IUGR) during the antenatal period to divert available oxygen and nutrients to the vital organs. During labour, with the onset of uterine contractions, due to the compression of the branches of spiral arteries, there may be a rapid development of hypoxia and acidosis. In addition, placental disorders such as infarction, villitis, vasculopathies and failure of trophoblastic invasion (e.g. preeclampsia) may lead to a reduction of placental pools resulting in utero-placental insufficiency (Table 2.1).

Fetal Response to Hypoxic Stress

In response to hypoxic stress, the fetus attempts to safeguard the positive energy balance of the myocardium to avoid myocardial hypoxia and acidosis. As the fetus, unlike adults, cannot rapidly increase oxygen levels by increasing the rate and depth of respiration, it decreases the myocardial workload by a reflex slowing of the FHR. This is termed deceleration.

Table 2.1 Causes of abnormal placentation

- Infarction
- Villitis
- Vasculopathies
- Failure to trophoblastic invasion (preeclampsia)

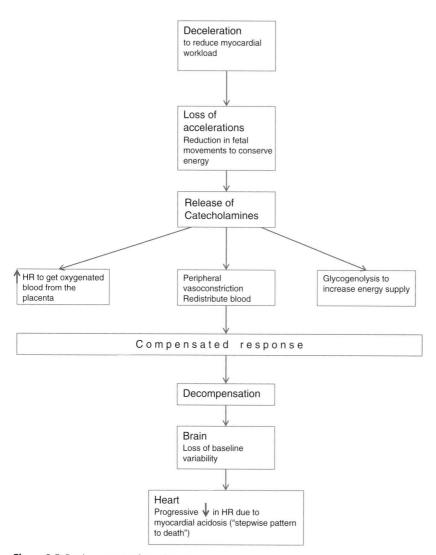

Figure 2.5 Fetal response to hypoxic stress.

If this reflex response to hypoxic stress is insufficient to maintain oxygenation of the central organs (brain, heart and adrenal glands), the fetus would conserve nonessential activity by stopping movements leading to a loss of accelerations in the cardiotocograph (CTG) trace. If intrapartum hypoxia progresses further, a fetus would release catecholamines (adrenaline and noradrenaline) to increase the heart rate, thereby increasing oxygenation from the placental bed and also causing peripheral vasoconstriction to divert blood from nonessential peripheral organs to central organs (Figure 2.5). In addition, catecholamines increase breakdown of glycogen to glucose to increase energy substrate to continue maintaining a positive energy balance within the myocardium.

This leads to a compensated response, and the fetus would continue to demonstrate a stable baseline FHR and a reassuring baseline variability (5–25 bpm), albeit with continuing decelerations and a rise in baseline FHR.

This is followed by the onset of decompensation in the central nervous system leading to a loss of baseline FHR variability followed by the onset of myocardial hypoxia and acidosis characterized by unstable baseline and a progressive reduction of the heart rate ('stepwise pattern to death').

Summary

Fetus is not exposed to atmospheric oxygen during intrauterine life and, therefore, develops cardiovascular, metabolic and haematological adaptation to ensure adequate oxygenation to central organs. In response to hypoxic stress, the only organ the fetus attempts to safeguard is the myocardium ('the pump') so as to maintain continued perfusion to other vital organs. A reflex decrease in FHR (deceleration), conservation of energy (loss of fetal movements) and release of catecholamines to increase placental circulation redistribute blood from peripheral organs to central organs and increase the availability of energy substrate (glucose). Failure in any of these mechanisms may lead to the onset of hypoxia and metabolic acidosis, leading to neurological damage or death.

Further Reading

1. Sadler T W. *Langman's Medical Embryology.* 12th edition. Baltimore: Wolters Kluwer/ Lippincott Williams & Wilkins; 2012.

2. Sadler T W. Third Week of Development: Trilaminar Germ Disc. In: *Langman's Medical Embryology.* 12th edition. Baltimore: Wolters Kluwer/ Lippincott Williams & Wilkins; 2012. p. 59–61.

3. Schoenwolf G C, Bleyl S B, Brauer P R, Francis-West P H. Second Week: Becoming Bilaminar and Fully Implanting. In: *Larsen's Human Embryology.*

4th edition. Philadelphia: Churchill Livingstone Elsevier; 2009. p. 51–68.

4. Carlson B M. Placenta and Extraembryonic Membranes. In: *Human Embryology and Developmental Biology.* 5th edition. Philadelphia: Mosby Elsevier; 2014. p. 120–129.

5. FitzGerald M J T, FitzGerald M. Implantation. In: *Human Embryology.* 1st edition. London: Baillière Tindall; 1994. p. 15–20.

6. Hardy K. Embryology. Chapter In: Bennett P, Williamson C. (eds). *Basic Science in Obstetrics and Gynaecology.* 4th edition. Churchill Livingston; 2010.

Chapter

3

Physiology of Fetal Heart Rate Control and Types of Intrapartum Hypoxia

Anna Gracia-Perez-Bonfils and Edwin Chandraharan

Based on the rapidity of evolution, intrapartum hypoxia may be acute (i.e. sudden cessation of fetal circulation), subacute (developing over 30–60 minutes) or gradually evolving (developing over several hours). Pre-existing long-standing or chronic hypoxia may occur in patients with preeclampsia or placental disorders, where the damaging insult takes place in the antenatal period. However, continuation of labour may potentiate ongoing 'chronic' hypoxic insult. It is essential to understand the features observed on the cardiotocograph (CTG) trace during different types of intrapartum hypoxia so as to institute timely and appropriate intervention to improve perinatal outcomes.

Physiology of Fetal Heart Rate Control

The fetal heart rate (FHR), just like in adults, is controlled by both autonomic and somatic components of the central nervous system. The former controls visceral functions and is composed of sympathetic and parasympathetic systems, which are constantly interacting with each other to increase and decrease the heart rate, respectively. The 'agreement' reached following this interaction is indicated by the *baseline* FHR. In addition, the constant fluctuation between sympathetic and parasympathetic nervous systems creates the 'bandwidth' of this baseline, which is observed on the CTG trace as the *baseline variability*. Somatic nervous system is responsible for voluntary control of body movements via skeletal muscles and it accounts for the occurrence of *accelerations* on the CTG trace. However, accelerations may also be seen in anaesthetized fetuses indicating that somatic nervous system activity may also be centrally mediated.

During labour, a fetus undergoes the most stressful journey of his/her entire life and will have to use all his/her available resources to adapt to the constantly evolving and rapidly changing intrauterine environment. Every fetus will have his/her own unique physiological reserve, which may be modified by a combination of both antenatal (e.g. pre- or postmaturity intrauterine growth restriction) and intrapartum risk factors (e.g. infection or meconium and use of oxytocin to augment labour).

Parasympathetic Nervous System

The parasympathetic nervous system is responsible for activities that occur when the body is at rest (such as listening to calm music, performing yoga). In contrast, the sympathetic nervous system is responsible for the 'fight or flight' response, which is essential for survival. The parasympathetic system will attempt to reduce the FHR in order to maintain a positive

Handbook of CTG Interpretation: From Patterns to Physiology, ed. Edwin Chandraharan. Published by Cambridge University Press. © Cambridge University Press 2017.

energy balance in the fetal heart in response to any hypoxic stress. This is because, unlike adults, a fetus cannot instantly increase the oxygenation to its myocardium by increasing the respiratory rate as it is immersed in a pool of amniotic fluid.

Parasympathetic activity is mediated by two kinds of receptors: baroreceptors and chemoreceptors.

Baroreceptors

These are stretch receptors found in the carotid sinus and arch of the aorta. During labour with the onset and progression of uterine contractions, both fetal head and umbilical cord may undergo repeated compression.

- Increased peripheral resistance secondary to the occlusion of the umbilical artery leads to an increase in fetal systemic blood pressure and resultant stimulation of these baroreceptors located in the carotid sinus and aortic arch. Once stimulated, the baroreceptors would send impulses to the cardiac inhibitory (parasympathetic) centre in the brain stem. This in turn inhibits the atrioventricular node situated within the heart via the vagus nerve to slow down the heart rate.
- In addition, stimulation of the baroreceptors also decreases the sympathetic stimulation of the heart. Such 'baroreceptor-mediated' decelerations will be seen on the CTG trace as *variable decelerations* secondary to umbilical cord compression. As these are generally short-lasting episodes related to uterine contractions, the fetal heart returns to the baseline quickly, and they do not expose the fetus to any hypoxic injury.
- Therefore, in the absence of other abnormalities on the CTG trace (unstable baseline or changes in baseline variability), the presence of early (head compression leading to stimulation of the dura mater, which is richly supplied by the parasympathetic nerves) or typical variable decelerations should be viewed as pure 'mechanical stresses' during labour. Hence, they do not require any interventions other than continued observation.

Chemoreceptors

- These are found peripherally on the aortic and carotid bodies and centrally within the brain. Chemoreceptors are stimulated by changes in the biochemical composition of the blood, responding to increased hydrogen ion and carbon dioxide accumulation and low partial pressure of oxygen.
- During labour, the activation of these receptors causes stimulation of the parasympathetic nervous system, which decreases the FHR. Nonetheless, unlike the short-lasting decelerations mediated by baroreceptors, when chemoreceptors are stimulated, it takes longer to recover back to the original baseline heart rate. This is because fresh oxygenated blood needs to reach the maternal venous sinuses to remove the stimulus to chemoreceptors.
- Due to delayed onset and recovery, they are termed 'late decelerations' and are often associated with fetal metabolic acidosis.

Therefore, decelerations secondary to the stimulation of baroreceptors will be in relation to compression of the umbilical cord and will have a sharp drop and a quick recovery. The duration between the onset and nadir of a variable deceleration is often shorter than 30 seconds and the total duration of the entire 'typical' variable deceleration should be <60 seconds.

- On the other hand, decelerations secondary to chemoreceptor stimulation due to metabolic acidosis have a more gradual fall from the baseline and take longer to recover to the original baseline FHR (at least a 15–20-second lag time to reach the original baseline). Therefore, due to their delayed recovery to the original baseline, they are called *late decelerations*.

Role of Sympathetic System and the Fetal Adrenal Glands

In response to persistent and ongoing hypoxic stress, fetal adrenal glands secrete catecholamines (adrenaline and noradrenaline) that have sympathomimetic activity. Catecholamines not only progressively increase the FHR, but they also cause peripheral vasoconstriction in order to achieve effective redistribution of blood to selectively perfuse vital organs at the expense of peripheral tissues and other nonessential organs ('centralization').

- Therefore, when interpreting a CTG trace, an attempt should be made to scrutinize for slowly increasing baseline FHR over a period of time to recognize fetal catecholamine response to a gradually evolving hypoxic stress.
- A baseline FHR of 110–160 bpm should not be considered normal during labour for all fetuses, and the baseline heart rate of each fetus should be used as his/her own control. For example, a fetus may increase the heart rate from 110 to 150 bpm due to catecholamine release secondary to ongoing, gradually evolving hypoxic stress but still be within the 'normal' range of 110–160 bpm.

The Somatic Nervous System

Fetal movements cause a transient increase in FHR, which is seen on the CTG trace as 'accelerations'. However, some studies have shown the presence of accelerations even after inducing fetal paralysis, and therefore, they are not always associated with fetal movements and appear to reflect the integrity of the somatic nervous system.

- Therefore, the presence of accelerations suggests the integrity of the somatic nervous system, and a 'healthy' fetus not only has sufficient reserve to supply to central organs but also has sufficient glucose and oxygen to expend on nonessential somatic activity. Hence, the presence of accelerations is a hallmark of a healthy, nonhypoxic fetus.
- A fetus attempts to compensate for ongoing intrapartum hypoxia initially by the onset of decelerations to protect the myocardium; the next step in the evolving hypoxic process is to conserve energy by reducing the movements of skeletal muscles. This will lead to the disappearance of accelerations on the CTG trace.
- In normal conditions, a fetus will have sympathetic and parasympathetic nervous systems constantly interacting with each other, which will define the baseline and variability in the CTG trace.

During labour, as a fetus is exposed to uterine contractions, a progressive intrapartum hypoxia may develop, which would trigger fetal compensatory mechanisms. Fetus will experience decelerations secondary to umbilical cord (baroreceptors) or head compression (parasympathetic stimulation secondary to compression of dura mater of the brain).

- Decelerations resulting from hypoxic stress will progressively become deeper and wider with continuation of labour.

- Moreover, a fetus will reduce its movements, and therefore, accelerations may disappear from the CTG trace.
- If hypoxia continues to increase, a fetus will secrete catecholamines that will progressively increase the baseline FHR to compensate for ongoing hypoxic stress by obtaining oxygenated blood from the placenta and redistributing this blood to essential organs at a higher baseline heart rate.
- If decompensation sets in, loss of baseline variability may be observed indicating hypoxia to central nervous system centres followed by myocardial hypoxia and acidosis leading to a progressive fall in baseline FHR ('stepladder pattern to death') culminating in terminal fetal bradycardia.

Features of a Normal CTG

Baseline FHR

This refers to resting heart rate excluding accelerations and decelerations. It is determined over a 5- to 10-minute period and expressed in beats per minute (bpm). A normal baseline FHR between 110 and 160 bpm is considered normal for a term fetus and if it is >160 bpm and persists for >10 minutes, it is called baseline tachycardia. This could be physiological in a preterm fetus (immaturity of the parasympathetic system) or be secondary to maternal pyrexia, dehydration, infection or rarely due to drugs such as betamimetics. Temperature can augment the effect of hypoxia on fetal brain and may predispose to fetal neurological injury.

In addition, a rise in baseline FHR can be seen as a fetus attempts to respond to hypoxia, resulting in fetal adrenal glands producing catecholamines. Therefore, as well as an absolute value, it is important to consider the trend over time; for example, although a baseline FHR of 150 bpm may be within a normal range according to the guidelines of CTG interpretation, an increase from a baseline rate of 110 bpm from the beginning of the CTG to 150 bpm needs to be taken seriously to exclude gradually evolving hypoxia (increase in baseline FHR is preceded by decelerations) or ongoing chorioamnionitis (usually increase in baseline FHR without any preceding decelerations). 'Complicated tachycardias', which are often seen alongside a reduction in baseline variability or decelerations, should be considered ominous. It is vital to compare current baseline FHR with previously recorded baseline during the last antenatal clinical visit or from a previous CTG trace to determine a rise in baseline secondary to a long-standing utero-placental insufficiency.

Similarly, a baseline FHR <110 bpm lasting >10 minutes is called a baseline bradycardia. Postterm fetuses may have baseline bradycardia due to the predominance of the parasympathetic nervous system with advancing gestation. Cardiac conduction defects (congenital heart blocks) can also result in baseline bradycardia. Terminal bradycardia may occur secondary to acute hypoxic events such as umbilical cord prolapse, placental abruption or uterine rupture.

Variability

This is a variation in the FHR above and below the baseline (i.e. the 'bandwidth') and reflects the continuous interactions of sympathetic and parasympathetic nervous systems. Normal variability of 5–25 implies that both components of the autonomic nervous system are functioning well, and therefore, fetal hypoxia is unlikely. Reduced baseline variability of <5 bpm

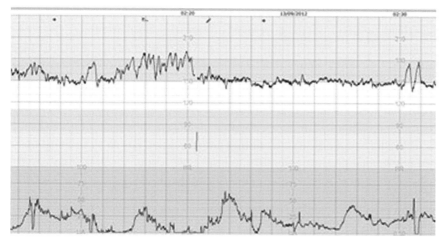

Figure 3.1 Normal CTG indicating the integrity of the autonomic nervous system (stable baseline FHR and reassuring variability) and the integrity of the somatic nervous system (presence of accelerations). In addition, there is no evidence of any hypoxic or mechanical stress (absence of decelerations) and presence of active and quiet epochs ('cycling').

may represent a quiet sleep phase or may indicate hypoxia to the central nervous system (together with an increase in baseline FHR and preceding decelerations). It may also be secondary to drugs (CNS depressants such as pethidine), infection or cerebral haemorrhage. Increased variability >25 bpm is called 'saltatory pattern' and needs further consideration as it may occur in a rapidly evolving hypoxia, especially in the second stage of labour with active maternal pushing. Therefore, an urgent action is mandatory to improve fetal oxygenation (stopping oxytocin infusion, stopping maternal pushing) if a saltatory pattern is encountered in association with decelerations to avoid hypoxic-ischaemic injury. If no interventions are possible, an urgent delivery should be considered.

Accelerations

These refer to a transient increase in FHR of 15 beats or more for more than 15 seconds. As discussed previously, accelerations appear to reflect the integrity of the somatic nervous system as they are usually associated with fetal movements. The significance of the absence of accelerations in the presence of a normal baseline and variability and the absence of decelerations has yet to be determined. The presence of accelerations, especially with cycling of FHR, is a hallmark of fetal well-being. Figure 3.1 illustrates a normal CTG trace with a reassuring, stable baseline fetal heart rate, a reassuring variability, presence of accelerations and absence of decelerations. However, the disappearance of accelerations following the onset of decelerations is a feature of gradually evolving hypoxia.

Decelerations

These refer to transient episodes of slowing of the FHR below the baseline rate, >15 beats and lasting more than 15 seconds. The decelerations have been traditionally classified as early (fetal head compression), late (utero-placental insufficiency) and variable (umbilical cord compression) in relation to uterine contractions. Nevertheless, during labour, more than one pathophysiological process (fetal head compression, umbilical cord compression or utero-placental insufficiency) may arise simultaneously, and therefore, decelerations may have different characteristics from the three standard types described below:

Early decelerations: True early decelerations are relatively uncommon in practice. They are a mirror image of uterine contraction, starting with the onset of contraction, reaching the nadir with the peak of the contraction and returning to baseline FHR at the end of contraction. They occur secondary to head compression often late in the first stage and in the second stage of labour. Compression of the head causes parasympathetic stimulation through the vagus nerve and a resultant deceleration of the FHR. It is believed that the fetus attempts to reduce its blood pressure by slowing down its heart rate so as to compensate for increased intracranial pressure secondary to head compassion. The presence of decelerations, which resemble early decelerations in early labour, should be viewed with caution especially if they are associated with a reduced baseline FHR variability, as head compression is unlikely in early labour and may be due to atypical variable or late deceleration that has been misclassified.

Late decelerations: Late decelerations are so termed because, in relation to uterine contractions, they occur 'late': both the onset of decelerations as well as the subsequent recovery to the baseline occurs after the beginning and after the end of a uterine contraction, respectively. The nadir of these decelerations is seen around 20 seconds after the peak of contraction, with the return to baseline occurring approximately 20 seconds after the end of contraction.

- Late decelerations are usually due to utero-placental insufficiency associated with fetal hypoxaemia and resultant hypercarbia and developing acidosis. This results in the stimulation of chemoreceptors leading to a drop in FHR. As uterine contraction ceases, the placental venous sinuses refill with fresh oxygenated blood leading to a gradual removal of the stimulus for chemoreceptors. This results in the delayed recovery of the FHR to its original baseline.
- In the presence of late decelerations and based on other features of the CTG trace and the clinical situation, an intervention aiming to increase the utero-placental circulation should be instituted.
- These interventions may include changing maternal position, administering intravenous fluids, stopping or reducing oxytocin infusions and use of tocolytics in cases of uterine hyperstimulation. If there is no improvement in fetal condition, an additional test of fetal well-being (i.e. digital scalp stimulation or fetal ECG) may be considered if it is intended to continue with the labour. In the presence of features suggestive of fetal decompensation (e.g. loss of baseline FHR variability) or further deterioration of the CTG trace despite intrauterine resuscitation, immediate delivery should be accomplished.

Variable decelerations: These are the most common type of decelerations, and approximately 80–90 per cent of all decelerations are variable decelerations.

They are so named because they vary in shape, form and timing in relation to uterine contraction. They are due to umbilical cord compression. Considering the shape and duration of decelerations, there are two types of variable decelerations, with different characteristics.

Typical or uncomplicated variable decelerations are characterized by a drop of <60 bpm, duration of <60 seconds and presence of 'shouldering', which consists in a slight increase in FHR both before and after deceleration. Typical variable decelerations are secondary

Table 3.1 Features of complicated ('atypical') variable decelerations

- Duration more than 60 seconds
- Drop of more than 60 bpm
- Loss of shouldering
- Overshoot
- Loss of variability within the deceleration
- Slow recovery
- Biphasic decelerations

to mechanical compression of the umbilical cord, and in the presence of normal baseline and variability, they may continue for a considerable length of time before fetal hypoxia develops.

Atypical or complicated variable decelerations have lost the 'typical' features such as shouldering. They can drop more than 60 bpm and last longer than 60 seconds. They can present with an 'overshoot' (an increase of FHR above the baseline following the recovery of deceleration and returning to baseline) or have loss of variability within the deceleration or may have a biphasic pattern. (Table 3.1 shows the features of complicated variable decelerations.)

Unlike typical variable decelerations, atypical variable decelerations are not due to transient umbilical cord compression alone.

They may be due to sustained and prolonged umbilical cord compression and may signify coexisting utero-placental insufficiency. If associated with adverse changes in baseline FHR with loss of baseline variability, it may indicate that the fetus is losing its ability to compensate for ongoing hypoxic or mechanical stress. It is therefore essential that the CTG trace is re-evaluated over time.

The importance of reviewing the entire CTG trace and considering the clinical scenario rather than just a segment of CTG trace in isolation cannot be overemphasized.

Types of Intrapartum Hypoxia

Based on the rapidity of onset, intrapartum hypoxia is classified into the following four types:

Acute Hypoxia

A single prolonged deceleration with a sudden drop in baseline FHR <80 bpm, persisting for >3 minutes (Figure 3.2). Such a sharp and long deceleration causes a rapid onset of metabolic acidosis if it occurs secondary to an intrapartum accident (placental abruption, umbilical cord prolapse and uterine rupture) and pH decreases at a rate of >0.01 per minute.

Recommended management includes:

1. Immediate assessment to exclude the three major 'accidents' during labour (cord prolapse, placental abruption or caesarean scar rupture).
2. Correct iatrogenic causes such as uterine hyperstimulation secondary to an excess of oxytocin infusion or maternal hypotension due to anaesthesia. Stopping oxytocin and considering administration of tocolysis (such as terbutaline 250 mcg subcutaneously) will help resolve uterine hyperstimulation, and the administration of intravenous saline bolus will help correct maternal hypotension.
3. Change maternal position.

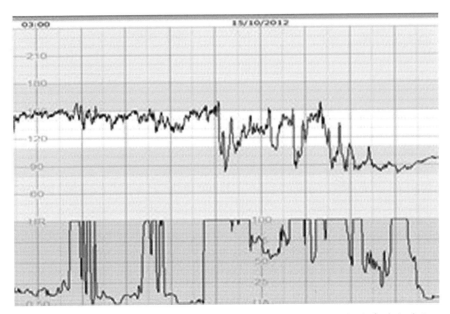

Figure 3.2 Acute hypoxia. Note the sudden fall in FHR due to an acute interruption in fetal circulation.

4. Assess the CTG trace seeking for *reassuring features*:
   a. Normality in the CTG trace prior to deceleration.
   b. Variability is maintained within prolonged deceleration.
   c. Signs of recovery within the first 6 minutes of deceleration.

   If these reassuring features are present, in the absence of acute intrapartum accidents, the likelihood of recovery is up to 90 per cent within the first 6 minutes and up to 95 per cent within 9 minutes.

   The '3-6-9-12'-minute rule – which recommends measures to correct iatrogenic causes by 6 minutes and to transfer the woman to the operating theatre by 9 minutes if there are no attempts of recovery, so as to commence an operative delivery within 12 minutes of the beginning of deceleration and to deliver the fetus within 15 minutes – is based on this principle.

   Considering the drop of pH of 0.01 per minute, a baby subjected to acute hypoxia after 15 minutes will have a decrease in pH of 0.15, which could mean, for example, a drop in pH from 7.20 to 7.05. In case of a fetus exposed to gradually evolving hypoxia through-out labour, its reserve may be already compromised at the onset of prolonged deceleration. Therefore, the resultant fetal pH will be even lower.

Subacute Hypoxia

It occurs when the fetus spends <30 seconds on stable baseline and decelerates for >90 sec-onds (Figure 3.3). Therefore, the fetus spends more time decelerating to protect its heart with only one-third of the time at the baseline to exchange gases and to protect its brain. The shortage of sufficient time for oxygenation leads to the development of fetal acidosis with a

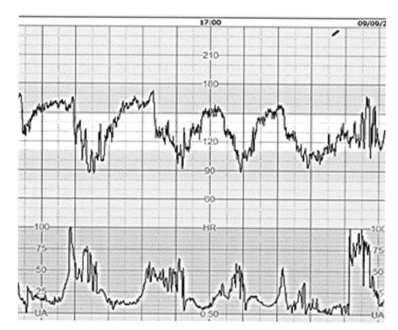

Figure 3.3 Subacute hypoxia: a fetus spends progressively less time at its normal baseline as compared to time spent during declarations. Also note the compensatory 'catecholamine surge'.

drop in fetal pH at a rate of 0.01 per 2–3 minutes. Therefore, the fetal pH may drop from 7.25 to 7.15 in 20 minutes. When subacute hypoxia is diagnosed, hyperstimulation with oxytocin should be excluded, and in case of active maternal pushing, suggesting the mother to stop pushing for a while may allow the fetus to recuperate.

Gradually Evolving Hypoxia

When a fetus is exposed to a gradually evolving hypoxic stress, it has sufficient time to mobilize its resources to compensate (decelerations → loss of accelerations → secretion of catecholamines leading to an increase in baseline heart rate (Figure 3.4) to redistribute blood to vital organs as well as to get fresh oxygenated blood from the placenta). If this compensation fails, then the onset of decompensation sets in, resulting in a decrease in perfusion to fetal brain. This will be seen on the CTG trace as a loss of baseline FHR variability. If no remedial action is taken, the myocardium will suffer a reduction in oxygenation with consequent acidosis that will be shown in the CTG trace as instability of the FHR baseline culminating in a 'step-ladder pattern' to death and terminal bradycardia.

Long-Standing (Chronic) Hypoxia

Chronic utero-placental insufficiency and antenatal insults may result in hypoxia persisting for days and weeks leading to attempts of compensation (increase in baseline FHR), chemoreceptor-mediated decelerations ('shallow' decelerations with late recovery) and evidence of decompensation (loss of baseline variability).

These fetuses would have reduced physiological reserves to compensate for any further hypoxic insults and, therefore, may rapidly decompensate with the onset of

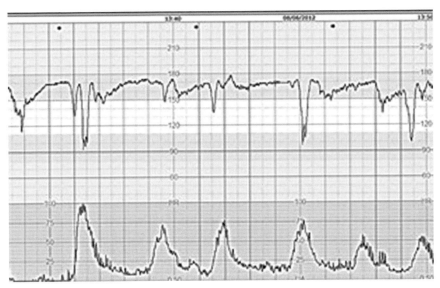

Figure 3.4 Gradually evolving hypoxia. Note the presence of decelerations, absence of accelerations and a rise in baseline FHR (catecholamine surge).

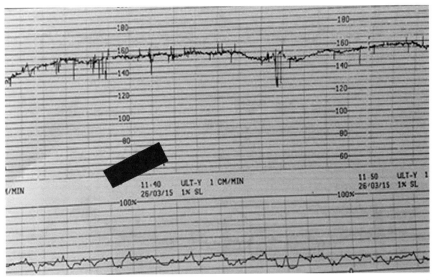

Figure 3.5 Long-standing hypoxia. The baseline FHR is in the upper limit of normal with a total loss of baseline variability and ongoing shallow decelerations, which are hallmarks of chronic hypoxia. Also note the total absence of 'cycling'.

uterine contractions leading to a progressive decrease in FHR (myocardial decompensation). Immediate delivery is indicated if features of chronic hypoxia are noted on the CTG trace (Figure 3.5), and if uterine contractions have commenced and immediate delivery is not possible (i.e. operating theatre is busy), tocolytics (e.g. terbutaline) should be administered to reduce further hypoxic stress until delivery is accomplished.

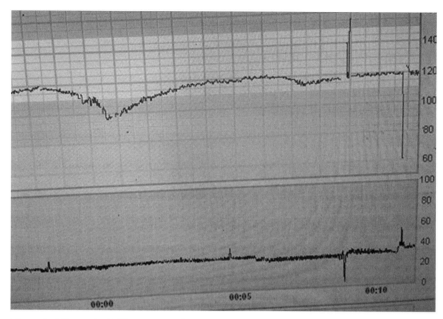

Figure 3.6 Preterminal CTG trace. Note the total loss of baseline variability with ongoing 'chemoreceptor-mediated' late decelerations suggestive of fetal acidosis. Unlike chronic hypoxia, this fetus is unable to maintain a higher baseline FHR to perfuse its vital organs, and due to myocardial acidosis, a 'wavy' baseline may be noted.

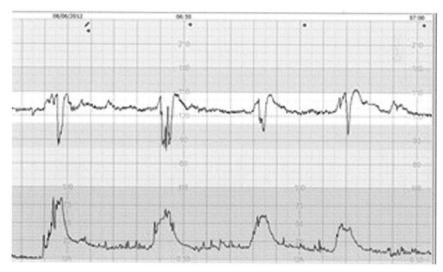

Figure 3.7

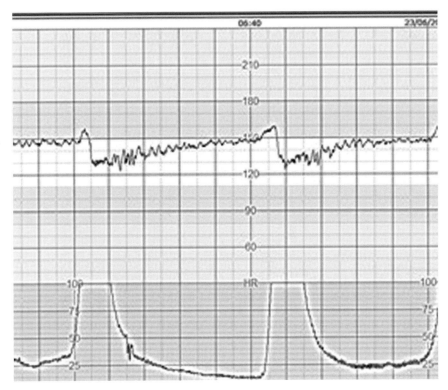

Figure 3.8

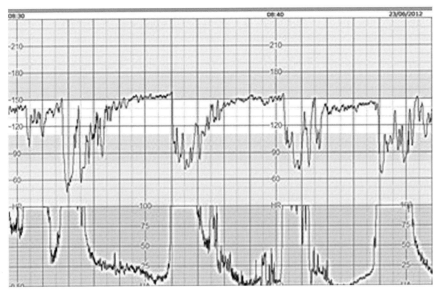

Figure 3.9

If baseline FHR is >150 bpm after 40 weeks of gestation, features of chronic hypoxia should be excluded.

Preterminal CTG

Once the fetus has exhausted all its compensatory mechanisms, a total loss of baseline variability and shallow decelerations would be observed on the CTG trace. Due to progressive myocardial decompensation, the baseline heart rate will progressively decrease (Figure 3.6) and terminal bradycardia may ensue, if delivery is not accomplished in time.

Exercises

1. How would you classify decelerations in Figure 3.7, 3.8 and 3.9? Why?

Further Reading

1. Chandraharan E, Arulkumaran S. Prevention of birth asphyxia: responding appropriately to cardiotocograph (CTG) traces. *Best Pract Res Clin Obstet Gynaecol.* 2007; 21(4): 609–24.

2. Williams KP, Hofmeyr GJ. Fetal heart rate parameters predictive of neonatal outcome in the presence of prolonged decelerations. *Obstetr Gynecol.* 2002; 100: 951–4.

3. Pinas A, Chandraharan E. Continuous cardiotocography during labour: Analysis, classification and management. *Best Pract Res Clin Obstet Gynaecol.* 2015; S1521–6934(15)00100-5.

Chapter

4

Understanding the CTG

Technical Aspects

Harriet Stevenson and Edwin Chandraharan

Introduction

The CTG machine (Figure 4.1) allows recording of fetal heart rate (FHR) and a representation of uterine activity over time. This allows an assessment of the integrity of autonomic nervous system control of the FHR (baseline FHR and variability), the integrity of somatic nervous system (accelerations), the sleep–activity cycle of the fetus as well as the presence of ongoing mechanical or hypoxic stresses (i.e. decelerations)

Parts of the Machine

CARDIOtocograph – Records the Features of the FHR

Transabdominal Monitoring – Noninvasive Monitoring

- The FHR is recorded both on the CTG paper and is displayed on the CTG monitor (Figure 4.2). It is also heard as an audible signal (which can be turned down or off as necessary).
- This is measured using a Doppler ultrasound device; this works by propagating a sound wave through the mother's abdomen. The speed at which a sound wave travels through a substance (or medium) is determined by the density, with sound travelling roughly four times faster in water than air.
- When two substances of different densities lie next to each other, the surface or boundary at which they meet is called an interface. As a sound wave travels through the first substance and comes to the interface with the other substance, some of the sound will pass or propagate through the second substance and some will be bounced back towards the source of the sound. It is this sound wave that is bounced back and detected by the Doppler ultrasound transducer.
- A Doppler ultrasound apparatus is placed on the maternal abdomen over the fetus' anterior shoulder (as determined by palpation) and repositioned until a good signal is achieved. A water-based ultrasonic gel is placed between the transducer and the woman's abdominal wall to provide a good contact. This ultrasound gel has a similar density to the woman's abdomen allowing sound waves to travel through it in a similar way, thus cutting down on interference.

Handbook of CTG Interpretation: From Patterns to Physiology, ed. Edwin Chandraharan. Published by Cambridge University Press. © Cambridge University Press 2017.

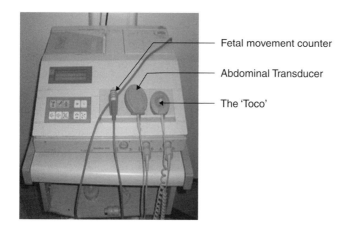

Figure 4.1 CTG machine with the transducer and the 'Toco'.

Fetal movement counter

Abdominal Transducer

The 'Toco'

- The transducer exists to make and receive sound waves. The sound wave is made by passing a high-frequency electrical current through a piezoelectric crystal. When an electric current is passed through a piezoelectric crystal, the crystal changes shape; this change in shape creates a sound wave, which propagates through the woman's abdomen. The piezoelectric effect is also such that when a piezoelectric crystal is squeezed or released from pressure, it will convert some of this energy into an electric current; this electric current from reflected sound waves is used to determine the FHR.
- How often the electric current to the piezoelectric crystal is turned on and off determines the frequency of the sound waves. Frequency is measured in hertz (with 1 hertz being 1 cycle per second).
- Doppler ultrasound in this instance is not being used to create an image of the fetus but rather to determine the frequency of the Doppler shift within the fetal circulation changes. See Box 4.1 for an explanation of Doppler shift.

Box 4.1 Explanation of Doppler Shift

In a CTG machine, the sound waves generated by the transducer normally 'hit' the fetal heart chambers, which are in constant motion, thereby creating a Doppler shift.

When a defined frequency of sound waves is sent from the transducer, if the surface on which they bounce off is stationary, the same frequency of wave length will be reflected back. In contrast, if the sound waves 'hit' a moving object (e.g. fetal cardiac chambers), then, the frequency of reflected sound wave will be altered resulting in a 'Doppler shift'.

Caution: Erroneous monitoring of maternal iliac vessels may occur. The Doppler shift caused by moving blood within the vessels may result in the maternal pulse to be monitored instead of the FHR.

Fetal Scalp Electrode - Invasive Monitoring

- This is an invasive method of monitoring in which an electrode is attached to the baby's head. For this method to be suitable, the membranes either must have already been ruptured or should be artificially ruptured to allow application of the scalp clip. There must also be sufficient dilation of the cervix to allow the electrode to pass through.

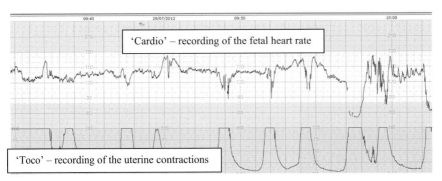

Figure 4.2 CTG display.

- Measurement of FHR is achieved by measuring the time between R deflections on the fetal ECG. This is referred to as the 'R–R interval'.
- One disadvantage is that this method of monitoring is not suitable for women with an increased risk of vertical transmission, e.g. HIV, hepatitis B or C. Rarely, the fetal scalp electrode (FSE) may cause injury to the fetal scalp.
- One advantage of this method is a reduced chance of 'loss of contact' as the clip is applied directly to the baby's scalp.

CardioTOCOgraph – Measurement of Uterine Activity

Abdominal Transducer - Non Invasive Monitoring

Abdominal transducer is used to measure uterine activity (tocograph).

- The 'toco' is placed on the maternal anterior abdominal wall over the fundus of the uterus, held in place by a stretchy elastic band to monitor the frequency and length (i.e. duration) of uterine contractions. The amplitude of the tocograph is related to the change in shape and tone of the anterior abdominal wall and does *not* reflect the strength of the uterine contraction. As the uterus lies beneath the anterior abdominal wall, it changes the shape and tone of the overlying abdominal wall during uterine contractions. This creates a pressure wave that is recorded by the tocograph (Figure 4.2).
- However, other factors can also change the shape and tone of the abdominal wall such as vomiting or pushing with the valsalva manoeuvre. Therefore, the recording on the tocograph does not always represent uterine activity.
- The strength of contractions is best assessed with how painful they are to the woman, whether she is making good progress in labour and whether there are ongoing changes (decelerations) on the CTG trace. Fewer contractions of a good length and strength can be superior to frequent, weak, short-lived contractions in achieving progress in labour.

Internal Pressure Transducers - Invasive Monitoring

- This method of measuring the pressure generated by contractions uses direct manometry or a pressure transducer on the tip of a flexible catheter, which is threaded into the uterine cavity via the cervix. Though, in theory, they offer more accurate measurement of strength and timings of contractions including the 'resting tone', they are rarely used outside of a research context in the United Kingdom. One of the drawbacks of internal pressure monitoring is that the uterine cavity is split into several compartments by the fetal parts. The pressure in different compartments will vary leading to erroneous results.

CardiotocoGRAPH– Display of the CTG Trace

- All CTG traces should be identified with unique patient identifiers and correct time and date as one would for any other documentation in a patient's notes. It is very important to check that paper has been loaded in correct orientation.
- One should be aware of the 'paper speed', which refers to the speed at which the CTG trace moves. In the United Kingdom, the paper speed is 1 cm per minute, and in the United States, a paper speed of 3 cm per minute is used, whereas in Scandinavian countries, a paper speed of 2 cm is used.

Paper Printout

- *Advantage*: It can be inserted into the hand-held notes and travel between centres with the mother. This allows any CTG traces done to be compared with the fetus' previous traces.
- *Disadvantage*: Paper traces are recorded on 'thermosensitive' paper, which degrades over time. This is a reason that traces are stored in dark-brown envelopes to avoid fading when exposed to light. For risk management, the CTG traces should be photocopied, which will avoid such fading and would enable storage of traces for a longer period of time.

Electronic Display and Storage

- Electronic display allows the CTG to be displayed both in the room and on a central monitor. This allows the labour ward coordinator or obstetrician to monitor the CTG trace of more than one woman at a time without having to go into the room or disturb the woman in labour. It allows the trace to be stored electronically on a central system for a prolonged length of time.

Pitfalls

Doubling of FHR

If the baseline FHR is <100 bpm, sometimes the CTG machine may double the heart rate and, therefore, an erroneous recording may be obtained. This would result in a 'bradycardia' of 60 bpm being recorded as 120 bpm, leading to false reassurance. A sudden shift in the previously recorded baseline heart rate, absence of accelerations and a reduction in baseline variability may give a clue to doubling of FHR.

Halving of FHR

If the baseline FHR is >200 bpm, the CTG machine may halve the FHR to 100 bpm as it tries to 'autocorrelate' the signals to ensure that the recording falls within the normal range.

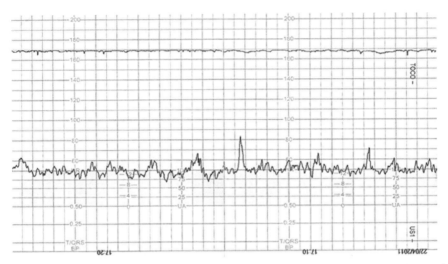

Figure 4.3 Recording of the CTG trace 'upside down' giving a false impression of 'reduced baseline variability'. Note the date and time printed upside down at the bottom of the CTG trace.

Therefore, in cases of fetal tachycardias, especially supraventricular tachycardias, a lower heart rate may be erroneously monitored

Erroneous Monitoring of Maternal Heart Rate as FHR

If the fetal heart transducer is placed over the maternal iliac vessels, especially during the second stage of labour when the fetal head (and the heart) is lower within the birth canal, the transducer may pick up stronger signals from the pulsations of maternal iliac vessels. This would lead to erroneous recording of maternal heart rate as FHR and resultant false reassurance and poor perinatal outcomes. A sudden shift in baseline FHR, accelerations coinciding with contractions and a sudden improvement in a decelerative CTG trace may indicate erroneous monitoring of the maternal heart rate.

Loss of Contact or Poor Signal Quality

This may occur due to incorrect placement of the transducer or due to maternal obesity. Internal monitoring using FSE should be considered, if there are no contraindications for the same.

Interference

The use of a transcutaneous electrical nerve stimulation machine for pain relief during labour may result in the interference of electrical signals, especially if fetal ECG signals are obtained via the FSE.

Incorrect Placement of Thermosensitive Paper

The CTG trace may be recorded upside down (Figure 4.3), resulting in confusion or errors in interpretation leading to poor perinatal outcomes.

Further Reading

1. Chandraharan E, Arulkumaran S. Prevention of birth asphyxia: responding appropriately to cardiotocograph (CTG) traces. *Best Pract Res Clin Obstet Gynaecol.* 2007; 21(4): 609–24.

2. Tolcher MC, Traynor KD. Understanding cardiotocography: technical aspects. *Current Women's Health Reviews.* 2013(9): 140–44.

3. Chandraharan E, Arulkumaran S. Electronic fetal heart rate monitoring in current and future practice. *J Obstet Gynecol India.* 2008; 58(2): 121–30.

Applying Fetal Physiology to Interpret CTG Traces
Predicting the NEXT Change

Edwin Chandraharan

Adult Physiological Response to Hypoxic Stress

All living beings are exposed to hypoxic stress in their day-to-day life and have inbuilt physiological mechanisms to compensate for short-lasting and long-lasting hypoxic stresses so as to protect the myocardium – the only organ that is protected at all cost. This is because, if the 'pump' (i.e. the myocardium) fails, every other organ in the body would also fail due to lack of tissue perfusion.

The inherent desire to protect the myocardium is exemplified in the anatomical arrangement of blood vessels supplying the vital organs. Coronary artery is the first branch that is given off, from the root of the aorta (where oxygenation is maximum) to supply the pump (i.e. myocardium). This is followed by the carotid arteries given off from the arch of the aorta to supply the brain. Therefore, these two organs have been prioritized from conception: the heart first and the brain next.

Adults are exposed to hypoxic stress during everyday activities, which include running, exercising, climbing stairs, sexual intercourse as well as brisk walking, all of which require increased distribution of oxygen and nutrients to muscles or sexual organs (i.e. whichever organ is active at the given time). However, if the heart muscle (myocardium) is forced to pump blood faster and with greater force (increased rate and force of contraction of the myocardium) without first ensuring adequate oxygenation of the myocardium itself, it would lead to myocardial hypoxia and acidosis due to increased oxygen demand.

Therefore, all living beings are inherently programmed to protect the myocardium first by maintaining a positive energy balance with the onset of hypoxic stress. This is to enable the myocardium to be well oxygenated (to maintain aerobic metabolism) prior to increasing the heart rate to supply the brain and other essential organs during hypoxic stress.

In adults, increased respiratory rate is seen as the first physiological response to any hypoxic stress to protect the myocardium from hypoxic injury. With the progression of intensity of hypoxia, both rate and depth of respiration increase to supply the myocardium, so that it could start pumping oxygen and nutrients to other essential organs, after ensuring a positive energy balance in the 'pump'. This is clearly evident during physical exercise, such as going on an exercise bike or treadmill, whereby the rate and depth of respiration progressively increases as the hypoxic stress worsens, and this is associated with tachycardia due to the release of catecholamines (adrenaline and noradrenaline).

Handbook of CTG Interpretation: From Patterns to Physiology, ed. Edwin Chandraharan. Published by Cambridge University Press. © Cambridge University Press 2017.

Catecholamines have three important functions: they increase the heart rate and the force of contraction of the myocardium to pump blood faster; they cause intense peripheral vasoconstriction to divert blood from nonessential organs (skin, scalp, gut) to supply oxygenated blood to central organs as well as a consequent increase in peripheral resistance thereby increasing systemic blood pressure to maximize the force with which blood could be supplied to central organs. Finally, they help in the breakdown of stored glycogen within the myocardium and other cells into glucose to generate additional energy substrate. All these physiological responses are aimed at ensuring compensation to ongoing hypoxic stress so as to maintain a positive energy balance within the myocardium, even at the expense of transient hypoxia to nonessential organs.

Fetal Physiological Response to Hypoxic Stress

A fetus has similar mechanisms to mount a physiological compensatory response to intrauterine hypoxic stress. In fact, its capacity to respond to hypoxic stress is greater than that of adults because of the presence of fetal haemoglobin (which has a greater affinity for oxygen) and the increased amount of haemoglobin (18–22 g/dL), which not only carries more oxygen but also acts as an effective buffer when there is respiratory or metabolic acidosis.

Unlike the adult, a fetus does not have the capacity to significantly increase the stroke volume (i.e. force of contraction of the myocardium) to the same extent and, therefore, increases the cardiac output predominantly through increase in its heart rate. In addition, a fetus is able to effectively and rapidly redistribute oxygenated blood to the central organs (brain, heart and adrenal glands) by shutting off blood supply to all the organs as the placenta performs the functions of the kidneys, liver and the lungs during intrauterine life.

However, despite all the additional protective mechanisms to deal with intrauterine hypoxic stresses, a fetus, unlike the adult, has a huge disadvantage because it is immersed in a pool of amniotic fluid. Therefore, a fetus is not exposed to the external environment and has no access to atmospheric oxygen. This means that a fetus, unlike adults, is unable to rapidly increase the rate and depth of respiration to protect its myocardium from hypoxic injury (and resultant myocardial acidosis) as its primary response to hypoxia. It is plainly obvious that increasing the heart rate to increase the cardiac output to supply central organs to avoid hypoxic ischaemic injury without first oxygenating the myocardium to maintain a positive energy balance would lead to a rapid myocardial hypoxia and acidosis, resulting in terminal bradycardia.

Therefore, the only mechanism available for a fetus to maintain a positive myocardial energy balance during periods of hypoxic stress that occur in utero is to reduce the demand of myocardial fibres because a rapid increase in the supply of oxygen by increasing the rate and depth of respiration, as in adults, is not at all possible. It is for this reason that the fetus slows down the heart rate (decelerations) during hypoxic stress in order to maintain a positive energy balance in the myocardium during episodes of hypoxic stress (Figure 5.1). This mechanism of reflex slowing down of heart rate in response to any hypoxic stress not only reduces myocardial workload and conserves energy but also improves time available for diastolic filling and coronary circulation. When oxygenation is restored (i.e. relief of umbilical cord compression or re-establishment of placental oxygenation as uterine contraction ceases), a fetus is able to recover its heart rate immediately to its baseline or even can increase it to a higher rate (due to catecholamine surge) to supply oxygen to the brain and other vital organs during hypoxic stress.

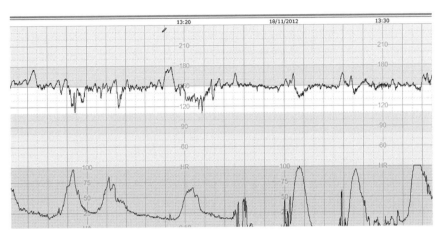

Figure 5.1 At the onset of hypoxic stress, a fetus may show decelerations to protect its myocardium in response to strong uterine contractions, while showing accelerations in between contractions. If hypoxia progresses, these decelerations would become wider and deeper, and accelerations may disappear as the fetus attempts to conserve oxygen and energy.

Deceleration, therefore, should be considered as a reflex fetal response to any mechanical or hypoxic stress to protect its myocardium. It is a useless exercise if one attempts to 'name and shame the decelerations' by using several terminologies such as 'type I', 'type II', 'early', 'variable', 'late', 'severe variable', as one does not do so for increased rate and depth of respiration that is observed during hypoxic stresses in adults. The morphology of the decelerations, similar to the rate and depth of adult respiration, would depend on the intensity and duration of the hypoxic stress. There needs to a paradigm shift in the reaction to decelerations, as there are not associated with fetal compromise but rather a fetal response to ongoing stress via a baroreceptor or chemoreceptor reflex mechanism. Some clinicians panic when they observe decelerations on the CTG trace, and this is similar to adults in a playground panicking when they observe athletes increasing the rate and depth of their respiration during hypoxic stress (e.g. sprinting).

Decelerations would be progressively wider and deeper as the hypoxic stress progresses during labour (similar to increase in the rate and depth of respiration in adults as the exercise becomes more strenuous). Similarly, decelerations would get shallower and narrower when the hypoxic stress is reversed (similar to a reduction in the rate and depth of respiration in adults that is seen when the treadmill is slowed down).

Instead of morphological classification of decelerations into 'early', 'variable' and 'late' and several 'unknown' decelerations, clinicians should classify decelerations according to three main underlying mechanisms:

- *Baroreceptor decelerations* occur secondary to an increase in fetal systemic blood pressure (occlusion of umbilical arteries during compression of the umbilical cord) and are characterized by a rapid fall in heart rate without any delay and a rapid recovery to the original baseline FHR (Figure 5.2).
- *Chemoreceptor decelerations* occur secondary to the accumulation of carbon dioxide and metabolic acids during hypoxia (utero-placental insufficiency, repeated and sustained uterine contractions or a prolonged umbilical cord compression) and are characterized by a gradual and slow recovery to the original baseline fetal heart rate even after cessation of uterine contractions (Figure 5.3).

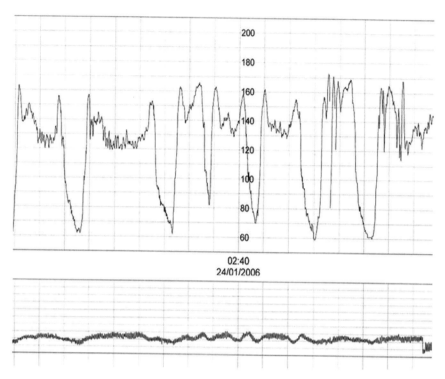

Figure 5.2 'Baroreceptor' decelerations with a rapid drop and a rapid return to baseline FHR.

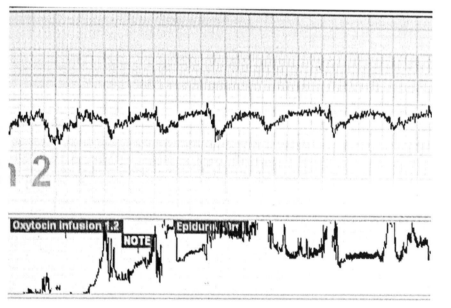

Figure 5.3 'Chemoreceptor decelerations' with a gradual recovery to original baseline FHR. The depth of deceleration is not marked as a baroreceptor deceleration and the heart rate continues to recover even after contractions cease.

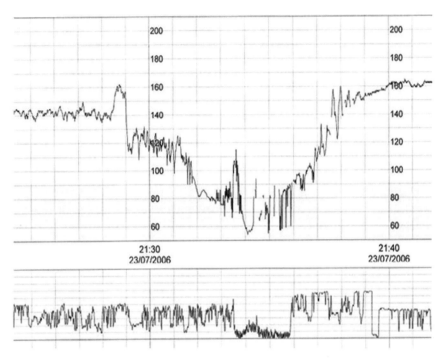

Figure 5.4 A prolonged deceleration. In acute hypoxic stress, a fetus rapidly drops the heart rate to protect the myocardium until the hypoxic stress disappears. However, in intrapartum accidents (e.g. placental abruption), irreversible myocardial damage may occur due to a combination of hypoxia and fetal hypovolemia.

- *Prolonged decelerations* occur as a reflex response to acute hypoxia (placental abruption, umbilical cord prolapse, uterine rupture or uterine hyperstimulation) or hypotension (epidural analgesia) to protect the myocardium from hypoxic ischaemic injury by reducing myocardial workload and to improve coronary blood flow (Figure 5.4).

Physiological Approach to CTG Interpretation: '8Cs' Approach to Management

Clinical picture: One should consider the presence of meconium staining of amniotic fluid, intrapartum bleeding, evidence of clinical chorioamnionitis, rate of progress of labour, presence of uterine scar, administration of medications to the mother or fetus, fetal cardiac malformations, ongoing uterine hyperstimulation and fetal reserve while interpreting a CTG trace.

Cumulative uterine activity: This refers to the frequency, duration and strength of uterine contractions over a 10-minute period. Unfortunately, the tocograph does not provide information regarding the strength of uterine contractions. Calculating the total duration of cumulative uterine activity (sum of frequency and duration of contractions in a 10-minute period) would give clinicians a better indication of ongoing uterine activity rather than solely concentrating on the 'frequency' of contractions alone, especially when oxytocin is used to augment labour. It is important to recognize that fetal hypoxia may rapidly ensue even if there are only four uterine contractions in 10 minutes but if these contractions last for 90 seconds each (cumulative uterine activity of 6 minutes). This is similar to having six uterine contractions lasting for a minute each in 10 minutes. Similarly, if the strength (tone) of contractions increases, rapid fetal compromise may ensue.

Cycling of FHR: Cycling refers to alternating periods of activity and quiescence characterized by normal and reduced baseline FHR variability. The presence of accelerations signifies a healthy 'somatic' nervous system. Although the absence of accelerations is of uncertain significance during labour, the evidence of cycling should always be sought while interpreting CTG traces. The absence of cycling may occur in hypoxia, fetal infections including encephalitis and intrauterine fetal stroke.

Central organ oxygenation: This is determined by a careful assessment of baseline FHR and baseline variability. Baseline FHR is a function of the myocardium (heart muscle) due to electrical activity of the sinoatrial node and is modified by the autonomic nervous system, various medications (e.g. salbutamol) as well as catecholamines. Baseline variability reflects the function of the autonomic nervous system centres, which are situated within the brain and, therefore, indicates the optimum functioning of these centres. An unstable baseline and loss of baseline variability would reflect hypoxia to the central organs (myocardium and brain) that would require urgent action to improve utero-placental circulation through intrauterine resuscitation (stopping oxytocin infusion, intravenous fluids, administration of terbutaline and changing maternal position) and to ensure immediate delivery if intrauterine resuscitation is not possible or appropriate (e.g. in uterine rupture) or if the measures to improve fetal oxygenation were not effective.

Catecholamine surge: A fetus exposed to a gradually evolving hypoxia would release catecholamines, and this will be reflected on the CTG trace by a slow and progressive increase in baseline FHR usually over several hours. It is vital to recognize this attempted fetal compensation to ongoing hypoxic or mechanical stress so as to take measures to correct any avoidable factors (stopping or reducing oxytocin or changing maternal position) to improve fetal oxygenation. If corrective measures are effective, the FHR should come back to its previous baseline rate. Continuing catecholamine surge is energy-intensive to the myocardium, and if timely intervention is not instituted, this may lead to a loss of baseline variability (decompensation of brain centres) culminating in a terminal fetal bradycardia secondary to myocardial hypoxia and acidosis.

Chemo- or baroreceptor decelerations: The presence of decelerations would indicate ongoing mechanical (head compression or umbilical cord compression) or hypoxic (utero-placental insufficiency) stress. It is important to determine whether the underlying pathophysiology is through a baroreceptor or a chemoreceptor mechanism. A slow recovery to baseline FHR reflects a chemoreceptor-mediated response. In contrast, baroreceptor decelerations are characterized by a rapid fall and an instantaneous recovery to the original baseline. It is vital to appreciate that the fetal response is determined in-between the decelerations (i.e. a stable baseline and a reassuring variability indicative of good oxygenation to the central nervous system as well as a rise in baseline suggestive of ongoing catecholamine surge).

Cascade: It is important to understand the wider clinical picture and type of intrapartum hypoxia (acute, subacute or a gradually evolving), and the need for additional tests of fetal well-being to confirm or exclude intrapartum hypoxia would become less if fetal response to hypoxic stress (a stable baseline and a reassuring variability) is determined prior to making management plans. Clinicians should refrain from merely classifying the CTG trace into 'normal', 'suspicious' or 'pathological' (or category I, II or III/normal, intermediary or abnormal) based on the patterns observed on the CTG trace without incorporating the overall

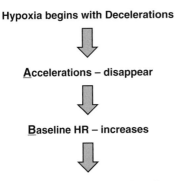

Hypoxia begins with Decelerations

Accelerations – disappear

Baseline HR – increases

Compensated Stress (Stable Baseline HR and normal variability)

Decompensation: unstable baseline and changes in variability

End Stage (Myocardial failure with a 'step-ladder' pattern to death')

Figure 5.5 'ABCDE' approach to predicting the NEXT change in the CTG trace due to an evolving hypoxia.

clinical picture and fetal response to stress. A pathological CTG with a stable baseline FHR and a reassuring variability often needs no intervention as opposed to a 'suspicious' CTG with total loss of baseline variability or with 'shallow decelerations'.

Consider the NEXT change on the CTG trace if intrapartum hypoxia progresses (Figure 5.5). If a fetus presents in early labour with a stable baseline FHR, reassuring variability, presence of accelerations and cycling and is exposed to an evolving intrapartum hypoxia, it will show decelerations first. These decelerations will become wider and deeper as hypoxia progresses.

As the fetus attempts to conserve energy (i.e. stops movements of nonessential muscles), accelerations will disappear from the CTG trace. This will be followed by a 'catecholamine surge' to compensate for ongoing hypoxic stress leading to a gradual increase in baseline FHR. Depending on the individual physiological reserve and the rapidity and intensity of hypoxic stress, some fetuses may remain in this compensated state (i.e. ongoing decelerations with an increased baseline FHR with reassuring variability). The onset of cerebral decompensation will be heralded by a reduction and subsequent loss of baseline variability, and finally, if no corrective action is taken, myocardial decompensation will ensue leading to a 'stepladder' pattern to death culminating on a terminal bradycardia.

Key Messages on Physiology-Based CTG Interpretation

- A fetus would attempt to protect its myocardium in response to a hypoxic or mechanical stress by slowing its heart rate to conserve energy and to preserve a positive myocardial energy balance. This reflex slowing of the heart is termed deceleration.
- A stable baseline FHR and a reassuring variability denote good oxygenation of central organs (myocardium and brain) despite ongoing late or variable decelerations that may result in a 'pathological' CTG.

- Clinicians should anticipate a progressive increase in baseline FHR following ongoing decelerations due to catecholamine surge. This indicates a progressively increasing hypoxic stress and fetal compensatory response to redistribute oxygen to central organs. Immediate action should be taken to improve intrauterine environment.
- If no action is taken, a loss of baseline variability or saltatory pattern (indicative of hypoxia to autonomic centres of the brain resulting in decompensation) or terminal bradycardia (myocardial decompensation leading to hypoxia and acidosis) may ensure.
- Deep decelerations which are short-lasting indicate intact fetal reflex responses to ongoing hypoxic or mechanical stress, while shallow decelerations in combination of a loss of baseline variability may indicate a depression of brain centres, and this requires urgent action to improve fetal oxygenation or immediate delivery, if the CTG is classified as 'preterminal'.
- The '8Cs' approach to CTG interpretation may help understand the wider clinical picture and fetal response to ongoing hypoxia, type of intrapartum hypoxia as well as evidence of decompensation.

Exercises

CTG Exercise A

1. A 32-year-old primigravida was admitted with spontaneous onset of labour at 39 weeks plus 3 days of gestation. On vaginal examination, her cervix was 6 cm dilated with evidence of spontaneous rupture of membranes. Clear amniotic fluid was draining and the presenting part was at the level of ischial spines. FHR was 128 bpm on intermittent auscultation. Four hours later, she was still found to be 6 cm dilated and, therefore, oxytocin infusion was commenced.

    Time to predict the NEXT change on the CTG trace:

   a. What changes would you expect to see on the CTG trace after commencement of oxytocin infusion if the fetus is exposed to an evolving hypoxic stress?
   b. If hypoxia worsens, what would you expect to see happening to the decelerations?
   c. If oxytocin infusion is further increased and hypoxia worsens, what would be expected to be seen on the CTG trace?
   d. What would you expect to see on the CTG trace?
   e. After the onset of cerebral decompensation (loss of baseline FHR variability), if oxytocin infusion was further increased, what is the next (i.e. last) organ to fail and what would you observe on the CTG trace?

CTG Exercise B

1. A primigravida was admitted with spontaneous onset of labour at 40 weeks plus 6 days of gestation. Oxytocin was commenced for failure to progress at 5 cm dilatation, 2 hours after artificial rupture of membranes. Clear amniotic fluid was noted and CTG trace was commenced. Apply '8Cs' on the CTG trace (Figure 5.11).
2. What features would you expect to see on the CTG trace if this fetus is exposed to a gradually evolving hypoxic stress?

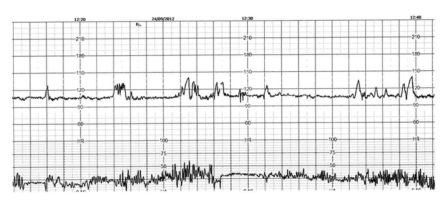

Figure 5.11

3. After protecting the myocardium, how will the fetus redistribute oxygen to central organs? What would you expect to see on the CTG trace?
4. What would happen to ongoing decelerations as hypoxia progresses?
5. What would you expect to see if there is onset of fetal decompensation?

Chapter 6

Avoiding Errors
Maternal Heart Rate

Sophie Eleanor Kay and Edwin Chandraharan

Key Facts

- The misinterpretation of maternal heart rate (MHR) artefact as fetal heart rate (FHR) can potentially mask abnormal FHR trace, giving the appearance of a falsely reassuring trace. This can lead to increased perinatal morbidity and mortality due to the nonrecognition of intrapartum hypoxia or fetal demise in the second stage.[1-4]
- The misinterpretation of MHR artefact can potentially appear as an abnormal trace, masking a normal FHR trace and resulting in unnecessary interventions such as caesarean section.[1,3]
- Studies have suggested that clinicians underdiagnose misinterpretation of MHR. The risk factors for MHR misinterpretation include an active fetus, twin gestation and obesity.[5] It is felt to be related to increased maternal movement in the second stage of labour.[4]
- External FHR monitors and internal fetal scalp electrodes (FSEs) are both susceptible to maternal artefact.[2,4]

Key Features on the CTG Trace

- During the second stage of labour, based on maternal physiology, one would expect MHR accelerations during contractions or bearing-down efforts, whereas, based on fetal physiology, one would expect the FHR to show decelerations[1-3,6] (Figure 6.1).
- Unexpected low range of FHR: Maternal baseline tends to be 60–100 bpm, whereas fetal baseline rate is 110–160 bpm.[2,3]
- Higher mean variability[1,2] with repetitive accelerations coincides with contractions (Figure 6.2).
- A sudden loss of FHR recording due to capturing the MHR periodically and then returning to capture FHR.[2,3]
- A sudden improvement of the CTG trace: disappearance of decelerations and appearance of high-amplitude accelerations with or without a shift in baseline FHR.
- Continuation of CTG recording after delivery.[1]

Handbook of CTG Interpretation: From Patterns to Physiology, ed. Edwin Chandraharan. Published by Cambridge University Press. © Cambridge University Press 2017.

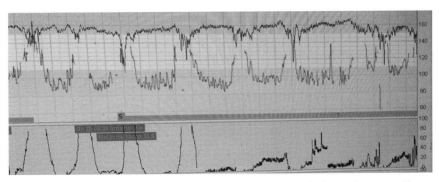

Figure 6.1 FHR showing decelerations with contractions (upper tracing), whereas the maternal heart rate shows accelerations with contractions (lower tracing).

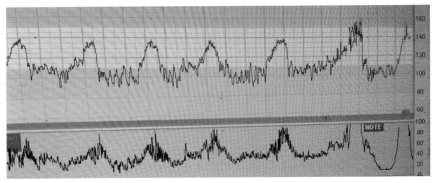

Figure 6.2 Increased baseline FHR variability with repetitive accelerations associated with maternal heart rate recording.

Key Pathophysiology behind Patterns Seen on CTG Trace

- The recording of MHR with external FHR monitors is due to the transducer picking up sound waves reflected from large maternal vessels.[1,2] During labour, as the fetal head moves deeper into the pelvis, clinicians often move the abdominal transducer further towards the pelvis so as to improve the 'signal quality' of the CTG trace, which increases the likelihood of picking up MHR.[2]

- FSEs detect and amplify FHR without the maternal signal. However, if there is no detectable signal, such as in the case of fetal demise, the maternal signal is amplified and displayed.[1,4]

- Normally with FHR interpretation, decelerations are seen with uterine contractions due to head compression, which activates the parasympathetic nervous system, leading to decelerations of the FHR, or due to umbilical cord compression or utero-placental insufficiency as a result of reduced placental perfusion.[2]

- However, if MHR is being interpreted, accelerations will be seen with contractions and active pushing. This is due to increased cardiac output related to increased cardiac stroke volume in labour, along with increased heart rate.[1] It is believed that haemodynamic changes occur due to the displacement of blood from the choriodecidual space and an increase in venous return to the heart.[1] Maternal anxiety

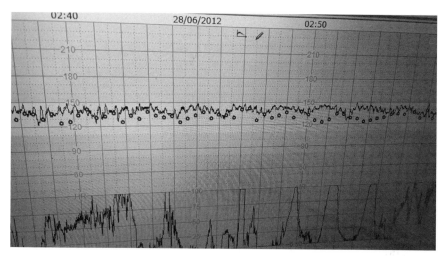

Figure 6.3 The maternal pulse (dots) is very similar to the recorded baseline FHR. In this case, the mother had raised temperature, and it is clear that erroneous monitoring was avoided.

and pain leads to catecholamine release during labour, contractions and active pushing, further increasing MHR.[1,2,4]

Recommended Management

- Once signal ambiguity is suspected, evaluate by assessing maternal pulse in comparison to auscultation of recorded FHR. If FHR and MHR are closely approximated, then it suggests misinterpretation of MHR.[3]
- Recording of MHR can be excluded by simultaneous recording of FHR and MHR such as by using a pulse oximetry probe.[1–4]
- Placement of an FSE is thought to reduce chances of erroneous recording of MHR, but it is still susceptible to artefact.[2]
- Fetal ECG signals can be analysed using a STAN (ST-Analyser) monitor with an FSE and 'reference electrode' on the maternal thigh.[2]
- If FHR is being recorded, then the ECG complex will show a p-wave. If MHR is being recorded, the p-wave will be absent because the low-voltage maternal p-wave does not have sufficient 'signal strength' to reach the maternal skin electrode placed on the thigh.[2]

Key Tips to Optimize Outcome

- The knowledge of the physiological differences between fetal and maternal heart rate ensures more prompt recognition of erroneous recording and appropriate action to ensure that FHR is correctly recorded.[2]
- Quick clarification and identification of concerns[3] is essential if the recorded pulse rate is similar to the recorded FHR (Figure 6.3).
- Simultaneous use of maternal pulse oximetry with FHR monitoring or STAN monitoring of fetal ECG waveform can help clinicians to exclude MHR monitoring with confidence.[1–3]

Common Pitfalls

- Late/nonidentification of MHR as FHR.
- Late/nonidentification of changes of heart rate from decelerations during contractions (indicative of FHR) to accelerations during contractions (indicative of MHR).

Consequences of Mismanagement

- Poor neonatal outcome secondary to missed diagnosis of fetal hypoxia, fetal bradycardia/tachycardia or fetal demise.[2,7]
- Inappropriate intervention secondary to interpreting MHR as FHR, with the background of a normal FHR.[1]

References

1. Sherman DJ, Frenkel E, Kurzweil Y, Padua A, Arieli S, Bahar M. Characteristics of maternal heart rate patterns during labor and delivery. *American College of Obstetricians and Gynecologists.* 2002;99:542–7.

2. Nurani R, Chandraharan E, Lowe V, Ugwumadu A, Arulkumaran S. Misidentification of maternal heart rate as fetal on cardiotocography during the second stage of labor: the role of the fetal electrocardiograph. *Acta Obstetricia et Gynecologica Scandinavica.* 2012;91:1428–32.

3. Emereuwaonu I. Fetal heart rate misrepresented by maternal heart rate: a case of signal ambiguity. *Am J Clin Med.* 2012;9(1):52–7.

4. Paquette S, Moretti F, O'Reilly K, Ferraro ZM, Oppenheimer L. The incidence of maternal artefact during intrapartum fetal heart rate monitoring. *J Obstet Gynaecol Canada.* 2014;36(11):962–8.

5. Herbert WN, Stuart NN, Buter LS. Electronic fetal heart rate monitoring with intrauterine fetal demise. *J Obstet Gynecol Neonat Nurs.* 1987;16(4):249–52.

6. Abdulhay EW, Oweis RJ, Alhaddad AM, Sublaban FN, Radwan MA, Almasaeed HM. Non-invasive fetal heart rate monitoring techniques. *Biomed Sci Eng.* 2014;2(3):53–67.

7. Hanson L. Risk management in intrapartum fetal monitoring: accidental recording of the maternal heart rate. *J Perinat Neonatal Nurs* 2010;24(1):7–9.

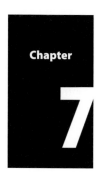

Chapter

7

Antenatal Cardiotocography

Francesco D'Antonio and Amar Bhide

Key Facts

Indications for Antenatal Fetal Testing

- The aim of antenatal fetal surveillance is to identify fetuses that are at risk of suffering intrauterine hypoxia with resultant damage including death. This includes each and every pregnancy, as no pregnancy is free of this risk.
- The goal of antepartum fetal surveillance is, therefore, to prevent fetal death and to avoid unnecessary intervention.[1]
- Several conditions pose additional risks to the fetus, thus theoretically requiring additional ways of assessment of fetal well-being. These conditions include prepregnancy or pregnancy-related maternal diseases and fetal-specific problems that may have a potential negative impact on fetal survival and development[2] (Table 7.1).

Current techniques employed for antepartum fetal surveillance include maternal perception of fetal movements, CTG, vibroacoustic stimulation and ultrasound assessment of growth, biophysical profile and fetal Doppler.

Role of Antenatal Cardiotocography

CTG is a continuous electronic record of the fetal heart rate (FHR) obtained via an ultrasound transducer placed on maternal abdomen and traced on a paper strip. Uterine activity is assessed using a spring-loaded device, which quantifies the extent of indentation of the uterine wall and is also traced simultaneously on the same paper. CTG is the most commonly adopted tool of fetal assessment before labour. It may be used in isolation or combined with other methods of fetal assessment, such as ultrasound and Doppler, as a part of fetal biophysical profile.[3]

Pathophysiology behind CTG Features

- The hypothesis behind the use of CTG is that the integrity of autonomic central nervous system (CNS), which primary regulates FHR, is a prerequisite for a healthy fetus.
- All those conditions causing hypoxemia and acidaemia may induce depression of the CNS of the fetus. This is reflected in abnormal features on the FHR trace.

Handbook of CTG Interpretation: From Patterns to Physiology, ed. Edwin Chandraharan. Published by Cambridge University Press. © Cambridge University Press 2017.

Table 7.1 Common indication for antenatal CTG assessment

Maternal, pregestational	Maternal, gestational	Fetal
Cardiac diseases	Preeclampsia	IUGR
Pulmonary diseases	Gestational diabetes	Infections
Renal diseases	Prelabour rupture of the membranes	Multiple pregnancies
Thyroid diseases	Prolonged pregnancy	Fetal anaemia
Autoimmune disease	Vaginal bleeding	Fetal arrhythmias
Hypertension	Reduced fetal movements	Oligohydramnios
Diabetes	Abdominal trauma	
	Previous history of adverse obstetric outcome	

- The mechanism by which hypoxemia and acidaemia induce an alteration on the CTG trace is not completely understood, but it is likely to be the result of the depression of the brain stem centres regulating the activity of the pacemaker cells of the heart.[4]
- Physiological conditions may alter the CTG trace. Fetal sleep cycle is associated with reduced baseline variability along with absence of fetal movements. It is a common cause of apparently abnormal CTG trace and may last for up to 50 minutes. Maternal administration of drugs that depress the CNS may also result in an abnormal CTG pattern.
- Accurate interpretation of a CTG trace should take into account the pathophysiology behind an abnormal trace. A fetus that is not suffering from a condition potentially leading to hypoxemia and acidaemia is unlikely to have an abnormal CTG on the basis of a pathological mechanism. Therefore, alternative causes should be investigated.

Interpretation of a CTG Trace

Correct interpretation of CTG requires a complete understanding of the basic features. These are represented by baseline heart rate (BHR), variability, accelerations and decelerations. It is important to remember that the knowledge of these basic features and the interpretation of CTG in the antenatal period are mainly derived from its use in labour.

Baseline Heart Rate

- BHR refers to the mean FHR over a period of 5–10 minutes in the absence of accelerations and/or decelerations and expressed in beats per minute. A BHR between 110 and 160 is considered normal. A BHR <110 bpm is termed baseline bradycardia, and >160 bpm is termed baseline tachycardia.
- Gestational age is the main determinant of BHR. There is a progressive decrease in BHR across gestation and should be taken into account especially when interpreting a CTG trace before 28 weeks.[5] The progressive reduction in BHR across gestation is thought to be likely the result of the maturation of the parasympathetic system.[6]
- Uncomplicated moderate bradycardia (defined as a BHR between 100 and 109) and moderate tachycardia (defined as a BHR between 160 and 179), especially in the absence of other abnormalities of the CTG trace, are not strong indicators of adverse neonatal outcome and have a poor predictive value for fetal acidaemia.[7,8]

Fetal Tachycardia

The main cause inducing fetal tachycardia is represented by maternal fever following infection, although fever from any source may increase BHR. Other causes of fetal tachycardia are represented by maternal administration of drugs acting on the sympathetic (terbutaline) or parasympathetic (atropine) system, fetal cardiac tachyarrhythmia (supraventricular tachycardia or atrial flutter), fetal hyperthyroidism and obstetric emergencies such as placental abruption.[7]

Fetal Bradycardia

Bradycardia may reflect the final stage of fetal compromise and impending fetal death,[9,10] especially in those conditions leading to severe fetal hypoxemia and acidaemia. It can also be associated with cardiac arrhythmias, especially complete fetal heart block. Short period of moderate bradycardia (BHR between 100 and 109, in the absence of other abnormalities on CTG trace) are not considered harmful for the fetus.

Variability

- Variability refers to the frequency bandwidth through which the basal heart rate varies in the absence of accelerations or decelerations. It is determined by the continuous and opposing influences of sympathetic and parasympathetic autonomic nervous system on the cardiac pacemaker.
- FHR variability is known to depend on several factors such as gestational age, baseline FHR, hypoxia, fetal sleep cycles and maternal administration of medications. Variability is sometimes further divided in long-term (LTV) and short-term (STV) variability. This distinction is valid for computerized analysis of the FHR. Such a distinction is impossible on visual interpretation, and the variability should be called 'baseline variability'.
- It is important to stress that reduced variability does not always represent an ominous cause. A careful assessment of physiological and pathological conditions leading to a reduction in CTG variability should be taken into account in order to correctly stratify the risk for the fetus.
- Reduced variability may represent an ominous sign for the fetus, predicting fetal compromise and eventually death, even in the absence of other pathological features on CTG trace.[11]

Accelerations

Accelerations are defined as abrupt increase in baseline FHR of >15 bpm and lasting for >15 seconds. They are usually considered a reliable indicator of a healthy fetus. The amplitude of accelerations may be lower before 30 weeks of gestation.

Decelerations

Decelerations are defined as abrupt decrease in baseline FHR. A deceleration is defined on the basis of its relation with uterine contraction, shape, depth and duration. Refer to Chapter 2 for details.

Sinusoidal Pattern

- A sinusoidal FHR was originally defined according to the criteria by Modanlou and Freeman.[12]
- Stable BHR between 120 and 160 bpm with regular oscillations.
- Amplitude between 5 and 15 bpm.
- Frequency of oscillations between 2 and 5 cycles per minute.
- Absence of accelerations.
- Oscillation above and below the baseline.
- A transient period of sinusoidal FHR may be present in a normal fetus, especially when it coexists with periods of normal variability. This is often seen during labour and is not associated with an adverse outcome.[13]
- A sinusoidal trace may be associated with various pathological conditions such as fetal anaemia due to red cell alloimmunization, fetomaternal haemorrhage, intracranial haemorrhage, twin-to-twin transfusion syndrome and ruptured vasa previa, medications, chorioamnionitis and umbilical cord occlusion.[12,14,15]

Types of CTG Examinations

Contraction Stress Test

- Contraction stress test (CST) is based on the response of FHR to uterine contractions and, thus, is a test of utero-placental function. The hypothesis behind the use of CST is that increased myometrial pressure following a uterine contraction leads to a collapse of the vessels running through the myometrium, decreasing the blood flow and oxygen exchange in the intervillous space. A healthy fetus is able to tolerate this relative reduction in oxygen supply. In the setting of utero-placental insufficiency, a compromised fetus is unable to tolerate the added stress and exhibits abnormal features on the CTG.
- Contractions are induced by incremental intravenous oxytocin infusion until a contraction pattern of three contractions in 10 minutes is established.[16] Nipple stimulation may also be used to induce uterine contractions[1] as an alternative. Observation of late decelerations following ≥50 per cent of contractions constitutes an abnormal CST. Relative contraindications of CST are represented by conditions that increase the risk of preterm labour: uterine rupture and haemorrhage, such as preterm prelabour rupture of the membranes, previous history of preterm birth, placenta previa and previous classical caesarean section. CST is largely historical and not used widely in clinical practice.

Non-Stress Test

- Non-stress test (NST) is one of the most widely used methods of antenatal fetal surveillance. The hypothesis behind the use of NST is that the heart of a fetus with an intact CNS responds to a movement with an acceleration of the heart rate (reactive or negative NST). NST is usually performed after 28 weeks of gestation and for a period of 30 minutes. The optimal interval between two consecutive tests is not clearly established and depends on the underlying maternal and fetal conditions, gestational age at examination and the results of the previous test.

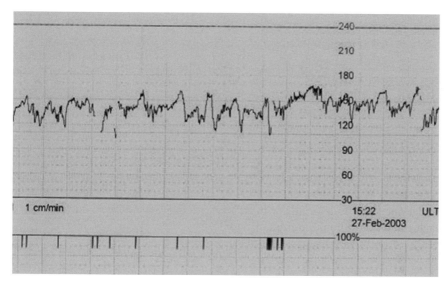

Figure 7.1 Normal antenatal CTG.

- The absence of fetal heart acceleration following fetal movement or absence of fetal movements is interpreted as a nonreactive or positive NST. The longer the time interval with absence of movements/FHR accelerations, the less likely that the explanation is physiologic variability.
- NST is a visual assessment and subjective interpretation of the FHR pattern. Several previous publications show that it has substantial inter- and intra-observer variability.[17-22] A reactive test is highly predictive of a healthy fetus; however, a nonreactive test does not necessarily indicate fetal compromise. False-positive rates up to 90 per cent have been reported in the past,[23] and a careful evaluation of the preexisting maternal and fetal diseases, gestational age at examination, fetal sleep cycles and maternal administration of medication acting on fetal CNS should be carried out when interpreting a CTG trace. NST is primarily a test of fetal function. A fetus that is acidotic is likely to have a CTG with abnormal features on the basis of a hypoxaemic mechanism. The first issue is, therefore, to identify those fetuses potentially suffering from conditions that may lead to hypoxaemia and acidaemia, such as IUGR. Ultrasound and Doppler assessment may help in this scenario.

The following parameters are widely accepted to be normal for the term fetus.[24]

- Baseline FHR of 110 to 160 bpm.
- Baseline variability of at least 5 bpm.
- Presence of two or more accelerations of FHR >15 bpm, sustained for at least 15 seconds in a 20-minute period[25] – this pattern is termed reactive.
- Absence of decelerations.

Figure 7.1 shows a normal antenatal CTG.

BHR variability and accelerations may decrease or disappear and decelerations in the FHR may occur when the fetus is hypoxic.[24] Figure 7.2 shows a pathological antenatal CTG.

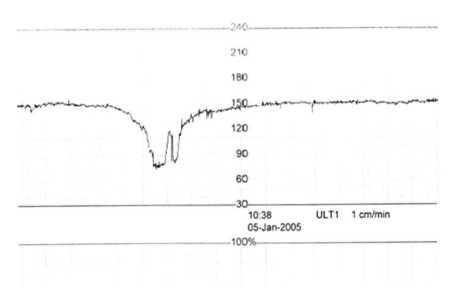

Figure 7.2 Pathological antenatal CTG. Note loss of variability and an unprovoked deceleration.

Computerized CTG

- CTG use is limited by problems with interpretation. Many studies have consistently shown suboptimal inter- and intra-observer reliability, potentially leading to unnecessary intervention or to lack of intervention when it is required.[17–22]
- A scoring system reduces the consistency of visual assessment but does not eliminate it. In order to overcome this limitation, computerized CTG (cCTG) is often used.[4,25,26]
- The CTG information is analysed by a computer to satisfy the criteria of normality over a period of 60 minutes, but the analysis can be stopped if the criteria are met before this time. These are called 'Dawes–Redman criteria' after their developers and are reported below.[27,28]

1. The recording must contain at least one episode of high variation.
2. The STV must be >3.0 ms, but if it is <4.5 ms, the LTV averaged across all episodes of high variation must be greater than the third percentile for gestational age.
3. There must be no evidence of a high-frequency sinusoidal rhythm.
4. There must be at least one acceleration or a fetal movement rate ≥20 ms per hour and a LTV averaged across all episodes of high variation that is greater than the tenth centile for gestational age.
5. There must be at least one fetal movement or three accelerations.
6. There must be no decelerations >20 lost beats if the duration of the recording is <30 minutes and no more than one deceleration of 21–100 lost beats if the duration of the recording is >30 minutes. However, no deceleration with an amplitude of >100 lost beats should occur at any time.
7. The basal heart rate must be 116–160 bpm if the recording is <30 minutes.

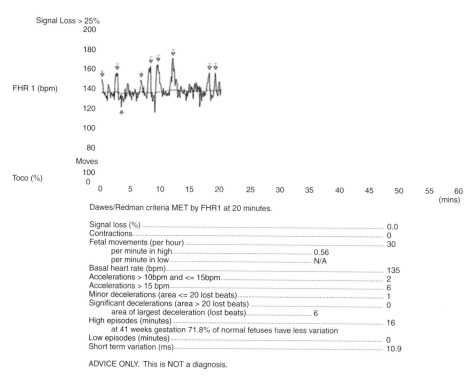

Dawes/Redman criteria MET by FHR1 at 20 minutes.

Signal loss (%)	0.0
Contractions	0
Fetal movements (per hour)	30
per minute in high	0.56
per minute in low	N/A
Basal heart rate (bpm)	135
Accelerations > 10bpm and <= 15bpm	2
Accelerations > 15 bpm	6
Minor decelerations (area <= 20 lost beats)	1
Significant decelerations (area > 20 lost beats)	0
area of largest deceleration (lost beats)	6
High episodes (minutes)	16
at 41 weeks gestation 71.8% of normal fetuses have less variation	
Low episodes (minutes)	0
Short term variation (ms)	10.9

ADVICE ONLY. This is NOT a diagnosis.

Figure 7.3 cCTG trace reporting the evaluation of Redman–Dawson criteria.

8. The LTV must be within 3 SDs of its estimated value, or (a) the STV must be >5.0 ms, (b) there must be an episode of high variation with ≥0.5 fetal movement per minute, (c) the basal heart rate must be ≥120 bpm, and (d) the signal loss must be <30 per cent.

9. The final epoch of recording must not be a part of a deceleration if the recording is <60 minutes, or a deceleration at 60 minutes must not be >20 lost beats.

10. There must be no suspected artefacts at the end of the recording if the recording is <60 minutes.

The risk for fetal hypoxia/acidaemia is extremely low if the Dawes–Redman criteria for normality are met.[28] Figure 7.3 shows a typical report of antenatal cCTG. Note that Dawes–Redman criteria were met at 20 minutes.

Pearls: CTG in Clinical Practice

• CTG is the most commonly adopted tool for fetal surveillance before labour. Indications for antenatal CTG include prepregnancy or pregnancy-specific maternal medical problems and fetal diseases, all having a negative impact on fetal development,[2] and CTG evaluation is recommended in all those situations, such as IUGR, potentially leading to fetal hypoxaemia and acidaemia that are mainly responsible for a change in normal FHR.[29]

• The main purpose of CTG as well as all antenatal fetal tests is to identify those fetuses at risk of suffering hypoxaemia and acidaemia in utero in order to organize prompt intervention.

Pitfalls

- Although it is widely used in different clinical conditions, the effectiveness of antenatal CTG in improving outcome for mother and fetuses during and after pregnancy is questionable. A recent Cochrane meta-analysis comparing no CTG with traditional CTG showed no significant difference in perinatal mortality or potentially preventable deaths, Apgar score or caesarean section rate.
- The risk ratio for using antenatal traditional CTG compared to not using one was 2.05 (95% CI 0.95–4.42).[30] This means that the use of traditional CTGs may be associated with a higher risk of stillbirth. Moreover, all the women involved in the studies assessed in this meta-analysis were at increased risk for complications. The use of antenatal CTGs is likely to do more harm than good in low-risk pregnancies, due to the low probability of fetal hypoxia. Computerized antenatal CTG was associated with significantly lower relative risk for perinatal mortality (RR 0.2; 95% CI 0.04–0.88) as compared to conventional CTG for fetal assessment in high-risk pregnancies, without any difference in Caesarean section rate. However, there was no significant difference identified in potentially preventable deaths (RR 0.23; 95% CI 0.04–1.29). Current improvements in ultrasound and Doppler allow reliable recognition of those fetuses that are at increased risk of complications.[31] Antenatal CTG may be of potential benefit in this group as an additional test on which to base clinical management. Moreover, cCTG looks promising in reducing perinatal mortality, and randomized clinical trials are needed to clarify its role.

Consequence of Mismanagement

- Antepartum stillbirth
- Hypoxic ischaemic encephalopathy
- Unnecessary operative interventions

Possible Future Developments

Adult cardiology literature has shown that mathematical assessment of variability of the heart rate is related to survival.[32] These investigators introduced a method called phase-rectified signal averaging (PRSA) that measures the variable elements in the signal, noise and artefacts of the CTG. The PRSA series can be employed to quantify the 'average acceleration capacity' (AC) and 'average deceleration capacity' (DC) of the signal. In the fetus, AC and DC are thought to quantify the activities of the sympathetic and parasympathetic nervous system. AC/DC have been reported to be significantly lower in IUGR fetuses as compared to normally grown controls matched for the gestational age.[33] PRSA is reported to perform at least as well as the STV on cCTG.[34] It is uncertain if PRSA will prove to be better than cCTG in the identification of compromised fetuses.

Conclusions

Conventional CTG is widely used for antenatal fetal assessment in the absence of robust evidence. There is potential for more harm than good with its use. Large inter- and intra-observer variability is one of the possible reasons behind this. cCTG has proven advantage over conventional CTGs, but the drawback is that it may not be widely available. The use of antenatal CTG to assess fetal well-being in low-risk pregnancies is not recommended.

References

1. American College of Obstetricians and Gynecologists (ACOG). Antepartum fetal surveillance. 1999. *Practice Bulletin* No. 9, October, Reaffirmed 2007.

2. National Institute for Health and Clinical Excellence. *Antenatal care: routine care for the healthy pregnant woman*. 2008. London: RCOG Press.

3. Lalor JG, Fawole B, Alfirevic Z, Devane D. Biophysical profile for fetal assessment in high risk pregnancies. 2008. *Cochrane Database Syst Rev*. 23;CD000038.

4. Dawes GS. The control of fetal heart rate and its variability in counts. In: *Fetal heart rate monitoring*. Ed. Kunzel W. 1985. Berlin, Springer-Verlag, p. 188.

5. Pillai M, James D. The development of fetal heart rate patterns during normal pregnancy. 1990. *Obstet Gynecol*. 76;812–816.

6. Renou P, Newman W, Wood C. Autonomic control of fetal heart rate. 1969. *Am J Obstet Gynecol*. 15;949–953.

7. Gilstrap LC, Hauth JC, Toussaint S. Second stage fetal heart rate abnormalities and neonatal acidosis. 1984. *Obstet Gynecol*. 63;209–213.

8. Gilstrap LC, Hauth JC, Hankins GD, Beck AW. Second-stage fetal heart rate abnormalities and type of neonatal acidemia. 1987. *Obstet Gynecol*. 70;191–195.

9. Jaeggi ET, Friedberg MK. Diagnosis and management of fetal brady-arrhythmias. 2008. *Pacing Clin Electrophysiol*. 31;S50–S53.

10. Larma JD, Silva AM, Holcroft CJ, Thompson RE, Donohue PK, Graham EM. Intrapartum electronic fetal heart rate monitoring and the identification of metabolic acidosis and hypoxic-ischemic encephalopathy. 2007. *Am J Obstet Gynecol*. 197;e1–8.

11. Smith JH, Anand KJ, Cotes PM, Dawes GS, Harkness RA, Howlett TA, Rees LH, Redman CW. Antenatal fetal heart rate variation in relation to the respiratory and metabolic status of the compromised human fetus. 1988. *Br J Obstet Gynaecol*. 95;980–989.

12. Modanlou HD, Freeman RK. Sinusoidal fetal heart rate pattern: its definition and clinical significance. 1982. *Am J Obstet Gynecol*. 15;1033–1038.

13. Young BK, Katz M, Wilson SJ. Sinusoidal fetal heart rate. I. Clinical significance. 1980. *Am J Obstet Gynecol*. 1;587–593.

14. Epstein H, Waxman A, Gleicher N, Lauersen NH. Meperidine-induced sinusoidal fetal heart rate pattern and reversal with naloxone. 1982. *Obstet Gynecol*. 59;22S–25S.

15. Murphy KW, Russell V, Collins A, Johnson P. The prevalence, aetiology and clinical significance of pseudo-sinusoidal fetal heart rate patterns in labour. 1991. *Br J Obstet Gynaecol*. 98;1093–1101.

16. Freeman RK. The use of the oxytocin challenge test for antepartum clinical evaluation of uteroplacental respiratory function. 1975. *Am J Obstet Gynecol*. 15;481–489.

17. Borgatta L, Shrout PE, Divon MY. Reliability and reproducibility of nonstress test readings. 1988. *Am J Obstet Gynecol*. 159; 554–558.

18. Donker DK, van Geijn HP, Hasman A. Inter-observer variation in the assessment of fetal heart rate recordings. 1993. *Eur J Obstet Gynecol Reprod Biol*. 52;21–28.

19. Flynn AM, Kelly J, Matthews K, O'Conor M, Viegas O. Predictive value of, and observer variability in, several ways of reporting antepartum cardiotocographs. 1982. *Br J Obstet Gynaecol*. 89;434–440.

20. Hage ML. Interpretation of nonstress tests. 1985. *Am J Obstet Gynecol*. 1;490–495.

21. Lotgering FK, Wallenburg HC, Schouten HJ. Interobserver and intraobserver variation in the assessment of antepartum cardiotocograms. 1982. *Am J Obstet Gynecol*. 15;701–705.

22. Trimbos JB, Keirse MJ. Observer variability in assessment of antepartum cardiotocograms. 1978. *Br J Obstet Gynaecol*. 85;900–906.

23. Devoe LD, Castillo RA, Sherline DM. The non-stress test as a diagnostic test: a critical reappraisal. 1986. *Am J Obstet Gynecol.* 152;1047.

24. Gribbin C, Thornton J. Critical evaluation of fetal assessment methods. In: *High risk pregnancy management options.* Eds. James DK, Steer PJ, Weiner CP. 2006. Elsevier.

25. Devoe LD. The nonstress test. 1990. *Obstet Gynecol Clin North Am.* 17;111–128.

26. Smith JH, Dawes GS, Redman CW. Low human fetal heart rate variation in normal pregnancy. 1987. *Br J Obstet Gynaecol.* 94;656–664.

27. Dawes GS, Redman CW, Smith JH. Improvements in the registration and analysis of fetal heart rate records at the bedside. 1985. *Br J Obstet Gynaecol.* 92;317–325.

28. Pardey J, Moulden M, Redman CW. A computer system for the numerical analysis of nonstress tests. 2002. *Am J Obstet Gynecol.* 186;1095–1103.

29. Nijhuis IJ, ten Hof J, Mulder EJ, Nijhuis JG, Narayan H, Taylor DJ, Visser GH. Fetal heart rate in relation to its variation in normal and growth retarded fetuses. 2000. *Eur J Obstet Gynecol Reprod Biol.* 89;27–33.

30. Grivell RM, Alfirevic Z, Gyte GM, Devane D. Antenatal cardiotocography for fetal assessment. 2012. *Cochrane Database Syst Rev.* 12;CD007863.

31. Alfirevic Z, Stampalija T, Gyte GM. Fetal and umbilical Doppler ultrasound in high-risk pregnancies. 2010. *Cochrane Database Syst Rev.* 20;CD007529.

32. Bauer A, Kantelhardt JW, Barthel P, Schneider R, Mäkikallio T, Ulm K, Hnatkova K, Schömig A, Huikuri H, Bunde A, Malik M, Schmidt G. Deceleration capacity of heart rate as a predictor of mortality after myocardial infarction: cohort study. 2006. *The Lancet.* 367;1674–1681.

33. Stampalija T, Casati D, Montico M, Sassi R, Rivolta MW, Maggi V, Bauer A, Ferrazzi E. Parameters influence on acceleration and deceleration capacity based on transabdominal ECG in early fetal growth restriction at different gestational age epochs. 2015. *Eur J Obstet Gynecol Reprod Biol.* 188;104–112.

34. Huhn EA, Lobmaier S, Fischer T, Schneider R, Bauer A, Schneider KT, Schmidt G. New computerized fetal heart rate analysis for surveillance of intrauterine growth restriction. 2011. *Prenat Diagn.* 31;509–514.

35. Modanlou HD, Murata Y. Sinusoidal heart rate pattern: reappraisal of its definition and clinical significance. 2004. *J Obstet Gynaecol Res* 30;169–180.

36. National Institute for Health and Clinical Excellence. *Intrapartum care: care of the healthy woman and their babies during childbirth.* 2007. London: RCOG Press.

37. Pillai M, James D. The importance of the behavioural state in biophysical assessment of the term human fetus. 1990. *Br J Obstet Gynaecol.* 97;1130–1134.

38. Henson G, Dawes GS, Redman CW. Characterization of the reduced heart rate variation in growth-retarded fetuses. 1984. *Br J Obstet Gynaecol.* 91;751–755.

Chapter

8

Intermittent (Intelligent) Auscultation in the Low-Risk Setting

Virginia Lowe and Abigail Archer

Key Facts

- Intermittent auscultation (IA) is appropriate for use in the low-risk setting where pregnancy and onset of labour have been uncomplicated. It facilitates the normal physiology of labour by allowing freedom of movement.
- The use of continuous electronic fetal monitoring in this group does not improve neonatal outcomes, but is associated with higher rates of medical intervention.
- When used cautiously, IA safely identifies the healthy fetus and promotes normality.
- Vigilance is needed in interpreting the findings to ensure signs of hypoxia or other indicators requiring investigation are not overlooked.
- This practice has been termed 'intelligent auscultation' to highlight the extension beyond listening for the presence of a fetal heart, but requires an understanding of fetal pathophysiology as well as the intrapartum hypoxic process and how this may influence the features of the fetal heart rate (FHR).

Recommended Method

- On first contact, there should be a thorough review of the whole clinical picture to ensure that pregnancy and labour have been low risk thus far. Enquiries should be made as to when fetal movements were last noted by the mother, and this must be documented.
- The fetal heart should then be auscultated with a pinard stethoscope or hand-held Doppler to determine the baseline rate. This is usually achieved by counting the number of beats heard over a period of 1 minute. The heart rate is recorded as an average number, not as a range. The choice of equipment reduces the likelihood of mistakenly monitoring the maternal pulse, and to reduce this risk further, the maternal pulse should also be palpated, measured and documented to demonstrate that they are different rates.
- Crucially, following this assessment, the caregiver has to establish fetal health. If fetal movements are currently present, auscultation of the fetal heart should reveal an acceleration of >15 beats above the baseline rate, demonstrating a nonhypoxic fetus.

Handbook of CTG Interpretation: From Patterns to Physiology, ed. Edwin Chandraharan. Published by Cambridge University Press. © Cambridge University Press 2017.

If there are currently no movements (although a report that these have previously been normal), consideration may be given to auscultation after stimulating the fetus by palpating the maternal abdomen or following digital scalp stimulation at vaginal examination. Again, an acceleration of at least 15 beats above the baseline should be observed.

- Finally, await a contraction and auscultate the FHR for 1 minute immediately afterwards to exclude decelerations. If there are any concerns throughout this assessment, then CTG monitoring should be commenced. This may be discontinued after 20 minutes if it is normal and there are no ongoing concerns about fetal health. In a low-risk labour with normal initial assessment, the fetal heart should be monitored for 1 minute following a contraction every 15 minutes in the first stage and every 5 minutes in the second stage.
- The baseline heart rate should be plotted on the partogram. If any decelerations are heard, or if a rise in baseline is noted, further investigation is indicated immediately.

Physiology behind IA

- IA should be the method of choice, where appropriate (i.e. 'low-risk' pregnancy), as it allows the mother to move freely, facilitating the normal physiology of labour. Furthermore, it avoids the use of CTGs in low-risk labour as the use of CTG in this situation may be subject to misinterpretation, raising the likelihood of unnecessary intervention.
- Accelerations demonstrate good fetal health as a reflection of an intact somatic nervous system (see Chapter 2). These may be associated with fetal movement or stimulation or may be spontaneous.
- Once chronic hypoxia has been excluded using the method above, then – excluding catastrophic events – for the fetus to become hypoxic, it will display decelerations and then a gradually rising baseline. This will be detected when following the principles of IA and a more intensive assessment of fetal health must be initiated.
- Quiet and active epochs ('cycling') are evidence of an intact central nervous system and will be apparent on the partogram.
- Evidence suggests that the type of deceleration cannot be established by using IA. By auscultating the fetal heart after a contraction, any decelerations heard will warrant further investigation. These will either be variable (cord compression) or late (utero-placental insufficiency/chemoreceptor stimulation) and will not have recovered by the time the contraction has passed. Decelerations that occur exclusively during contractions are not usually associated with poor neonatal outcomes.
- FHR changes unrelated to hypoxia may also be detected. An evolving tachycardia driven by infection, maternal pyrexia or dehydration will be visible on the partogram. Again, immediate assessment is required, including CTG analysis.

Pitfalls

- A thorough initial assessment is needed to exclude any conditions that may increase the likelihood of hypoxia developing in the fetus. IA is not appropriate in these cases.
- FHR must always be recorded as a single average figure, not a range. This allows trends to be seen clearly on the partogram.

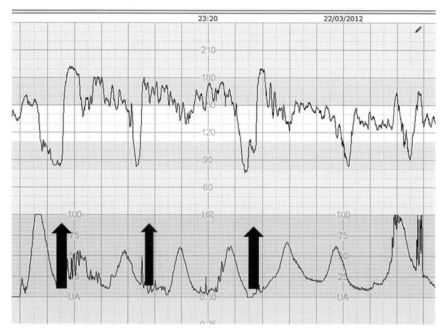

Figure 8.1 FHR 'overshoots', which will be noted as repeated 'accelerations' after each uterine contraction (arrows) during IA. Continuous electronic FHR recording should be initiated to exclude ongoing atypical variable decelerations suggestive of repeated and sustained compression of the umbilical cord.

- The fetal heart must be auscultated *immediately* following a contraction. Any delay may mean that the window of opportunity to hear decelerations may be missed, therefore failing to identify the first evidence of hypoxia.
- Baseline rate and the presence of accelerations and decelerations can be correctly identified using IA. There is, however, no evidence that either types of deceleration or variability can be identified. This is not a weakness of IA: the parameters necessary to highlight the fetus requiring further assessment can be detected. If the caregiver is attempting to monitor variability through IA, they have misinterpreted the principles of physiology-based interpretation.
- Accelerations after a contraction are physiologically unlikely, especially as labour progresses, and are more likely to be an 'overshoot' following a deceleration (Figure 8.1) requiring further investigation. This is because 'overshoots' denote an exaggerated fetal compensatory response to fetal hypotension secondary to sustained compression of the umbilical cord.
- A rising baseline heart rate warrants a thorough exploration of possible causes, regardless of whether this is an absolute or relative tachycardia (consider gradually evolving hypoxia where decelerations may not have been heard with IA or inflammatory/infective processes).
- Monitoring in the second stage of labour is more frequent due to the increasing stressors present. However, great care must be taken to ensure monitoring is accurate; descent of the fetal head means that the likelihood of mistakenly locating blood flow in the maternal iliac vessels is increased. Active second stage is also a time when maternal

heart rate (MHR) is often increased due to exertion; so misinterpretation is possible and caregivers must remain vigilant.

Exercises

1. A 30-year-old primigravida presented with spontaneous labour at 39 weeks, having had a low-risk pregnancy. On vaginal examination, cervix was 6 cm dilated, fully effaced with the presenting part 2 to the ischial spines. Bulging membranes were felt. She is requesting entonox for analgesia.

    a. Is CTG monitoring indicated? Why?
    b. On auscultation of the fetal heart, for 1 minute after the contraction, the heart rate is heard at an average of 140 bpm. Using the principles of IA, what is your diagnosis? What other information do you need?
    c. What is your action plan following assessment?
    d. Before the next vaginal examination was due, decelerations were heard using a hand-held Doppler following a contraction. What would your actions be?

2. Having had a low-risk pregnancy, with normal scans, a 25-year-old primigravida presented with spontaneous labour at 41 weeks and 2 days. Spontaneous rupture of membranes was confirmed on speculum 14 hours ago. On vaginal examination, cervix was found to be 5 cm dilated, fully effaced, and well applied to the fetal head, with the presenting part 2 to the ischial spines. Clear liquor is noted.

    a. On auscultation of FHR for 1 minute after a contraction, the fetal heart is heard at a rate of 150 bpm. What other information do you need?
    b. What are the possible causes of the findings?
    c. Is CTG monitoring indicated? Why?

Further Reading

Alfirevic Z, Devane D, Gyte G. Continuous cardiotocography (CTG) as a form of electronic fetal monitoring (EFM) for fetal assessment during labour. *Cochrane Database of Systematic Rev.* 2013;5:CD006066

Gibb D, Arulkumaran S. (eds) *Fetal monitoring in practice*. 3rd edition. Edinburgh: Elsevier, 2008.

Lowe V, Harding C. Intermittent auscultation. In: Arulkumaran S, Tank J, Haththotuwa R, Tank P (eds). *Antenatal and intrapartum fetal surveillance*. Orient Black Swan, 2013.

National Institute for Health and Clinical Excellence. Clinical guideline number 190 intrapartum care December 2014 www.nice.org.uk/guidance/cg190/resources/guidance-intrapartum-care-care-of-healthy-women-and-their-babies-during-childbirth-pdf (accessed 1 April 2015).

Schifrin BS, Amsel J, Burdorf G. The accuracy of auscultatory detection of fetal cardiac decelerations: a computer simulation. *Am J Obstet Gynecol.* 1992;166:566–76.

Westgate JA, Wibbens B, Bennet L, Wassink G, Parer J, Gunn AJ. The intrapartum deceleration in center stage: a physiologic approach to the interpretation of fetal heart rate changes in labor. *Am J Obstet Gynecol.* 2007;197:e1-236.e11.

Current Scientific Evidence on CTG

Ana Piñas Carrillo and Edwin Chandraharan

Key Facts

- CTG has been used since the 1960s. It was introduced as a method of intrapartum fetal monitoring in high-risk pregnancies to improve neonatal outcomes and to avoid long-term neurological sequelae. However, the rates of perinatal deaths, hypoxic encephalopathy and cerebral palsy have remained stable, whereas the rate of operative deliveries among fetuses monitored using CTG has been continuously increasing.
- CTG interpretation, which has been based on pattern recognition, has a poor positive predictive value for intrapartum hypoxia and a high false-positive rate. Only about 40–60 per cent fetuses with a CTG classified as abnormal by NICE guidelines have evidence of metabolic acidosis at birth.

Current Evidence

- The latest Cochrane Review, published in 2013, included 13 trials (>37,000 women). However, only two of these trials were considered of high quality.
- The use of continuous intrapartum CTG monitoring showed no significant difference in overall perinatal mortality rate. It showed a 50 per cent reduction in neonatal seizures; however, this did not translate to any long-term benefit such as a significant reduction in cerebral palsy.
- Continuous CTG monitoring showed a significant increase in operative deliveries, both caesarean sections and instrumental deliveries.
- The use of additional tests such as fetal blood sampling did not change the long-term outcomes but increased the rate of operative deliveries.
- Some individual studies (e.g. Vintzelios et al.) have suggested that the use of CTG may help improve perinatal outcomes.

Interpretation of Current Evidence

- To measure rare outcomes such as perinatal deaths and cerebral palsy (incidence 2/ 1,000), large number of babies need to be recruited to reach scientific conclusions.
- It is estimated that 80,000 women need to be enrolled in a study to achieve the 'power of the rest' to reach conclusions with regard to the reduction in cerebral palsy and

Handbook of CTG Interpretation: From Patterns to Physiology, ed. Edwin Chandraharan. Published by Cambridge University Press. © Cambridge University Press 2017.

perinatal deaths. So far, Cochrane Review has analysed only 37,000 women, and only two of the trials were of high quality.

- Earlier clinical trials on CTG and intermittent auscultation were heterogeneous with different cut-off values to determine neonatal outcomes and different criteria for 'pathological' CTG traces.

- There has been a continuous improvement in both obstetric and neonatal care since the CTG was introduced into clinical practice. Therefore, the older trials, which showed no evidence of benefit, may not be applicable in current obstetric practice.

- There were over 25 different clinical guidelines, each employing different classification systems and indications for continuous, electronic fetal heart rate (FHR) monitoring until the mid-1980s. Therefore, the older clinical trials did not use standardized criteria for continuous, electronic FHR monitoring.

- The largest randomized controlled trial, 'The Dublin Trial', that compared intermittent auscultation versus continuous, electronic FHR monitoring used fetal scalp blood sampling on both arms, which is not an accepted clinical practice. In addition, artificial rupture of membranes was performed at 1 cm dilatation of the cervix to exclude meconium staining of liquor in the 'intermittent monitoring group', which is also not an accepted clinical practice. Therefore, the findings of the Cochrane Review, which have been skewed by this largest randomized trial on intermittent auscultation versus CTG, should be used with caution in 2015.

- It is also very important to appreciate that earlier studies purely used 'pattern recognition' to classify CTGs without considering fetal physiological response to hypoxic stress. It has been well known that 'pattern recognition' is associated with significant inter- and intra-observer variability. Therefore, the reported increase in operative interventions may be secondary to overreaction to observed patterns. Conversely, a lack of understanding of pathophysiology of CTG and features of fetal decompensation may have resulted in poor perinatal outcomes.

- Therefore, it is hoped that the use of fetal physiology while interpreting CTG traces and timely and appropriate action when features of fetal decompensation are observed on the CTG while using intrauterine resuscitation to improve fetal intrauterine environment may help improve perinatal outcomes while reducing unnecessary operative interventions.

Future Developments

- There are two large multicentre randomized controlled trials ('INFANT' trial and 'CisPorto' trial) on electronic FHR monitoring which have been recently completed and the results are awaited. It is hoped that these will further increase the number of 'high-quality' evidence to appropriate conclusion with regard to the benefits of using CTG monitoring during labour. Whilst these studies have not yet published in Journals, the outcomes presented at International Scientific Meetings in 2016 by the authors of these studies suggest that the use of computerised CTGs did not improve perinatal outcomes.

- The use of fetal physiology (features of central organ oxygenation and of decompensation), types of intrapartum hypoxia and additional tests of fetal well-being that determine oxygenation of central organs (e.g. fetal ECG or STAN) may help improve perinatal outcomes without increasing unnecessary operative interventions.

Further Reading

1. Alfirevic Z, Devane D, Gyte GML.
    Continuous cardiotocography (CTG) as a
    form of electronic fetal monitoring (EFM)
    for fetal assessment during labor. *Cochrane
    Database Syst Rev.* 2013; 5: CD006066.

2. Chen HY, Chauhan S, Ananth C,
    Vintzileos A, Abuhamad A. Electronic fetal
    heart rate monitoring and its relationship
    to neonatal and infant mortality in the
    United States. *Am J Obstet Gynecol.* 2011;
    204: e1–10.

3. Donker D, van Geijn H, Hasman A.
    Interobserver variation in the assessment
    of fetal heart rate recordings. *Eur J Obstet
    Gynecol Reprod Biol.* 1993; 52: 21–28.

4. Macdonald D, Grant A, Sheridan-Pereira
    M, Boylan P, Chalmers I. The Dublin
    randomized controlled trial of intrapartum
    fetal heart rate monitoring. *Am J Obstet
    Gynecol.* 1985; 152: 524–39.

5. Khangura T, Chandraharan, E. Electronic
    fetal heart rate monitoring: the future.
    Curr Women's Health Rev. 2013; 9: 169–74.

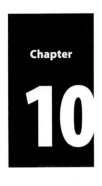

Chapter

10

Role of Uterine Contractions and Intrapartum Reoxygenation Ratio

Sadia Muhammad and Edwin Chandraharan

Key Facts

- The frequency, duration and strength of uterine contractions should be considered whilst interpreting Cardiotocograph.[1-3] During labour, uterine contractions compress spiral arteries and thereby interrupt blood flow to intervillous space leading to a reduction in placental perfusion.[4-6] Intrauterine pressure during labour may reach 85–90 mm Hg, and this is further elevated with maternal pushing. The Ferguson reflex at full dilatation of cervix further releases oxytocin, which increases the strength, frequency and duration of contractions affecting further gaseous exchange during second stage of labour.

- The onset of maternal pushing (active second stage of labour) decreases maternal oxygenation leading to a reduction in the oxygenation of placental venous sinuses and thereby further increasing the risk of acidaemia with higher levels of lactic acid and CO_2. Uterine hyperstimulation secondary to the use of oxytocin infusion during second stage of labour may further increase the risk of acidaemia as further reduction in utero-placental perfusion.[5]

- Most healthy fetuses cope with ongoing stress of labour without sustaining any hypoxic injury and are vigorous at birth. However, the use of uterotonics for induction or augmentation of labour leads to an increase in uterine activity. Scientific research suggests that when uterine contractions occur at intervals of <2 to 3 minutes, there is an increased likelihood of diminution of blood flow to intervillous space. If this is repeated, intermittent interruption of fetal oxygenation exceeds a critical level, then fetal decompensation may ensue and progression from hypoxaemia to hypoxia, acidaemia to acidosis and even asphyxia and resultant abnormal FHR pattern may occur.[7]

- Research comparing the effect of excessive uterine activity on the fetal oxygen saturation using near–infra red spectrometry concluded that fetal cerebral oxygen saturation reached the lowest level of 92 seconds after the peak of contraction with approximately 90 seconds to return to original baseline level.[8] In addition, an incomplete recovery to baseline was observed when uterine contractions occurred once in every 2 minutes and fetal oxygen saturation decreased incrementally after each contraction recovering only after oxytocin was stopped.

Handbook of CTG Interpretation: From Patterns to Physiology, ed. Edwin Chandraharan. Published by Cambridge University Press. © Cambridge University Press 2017.

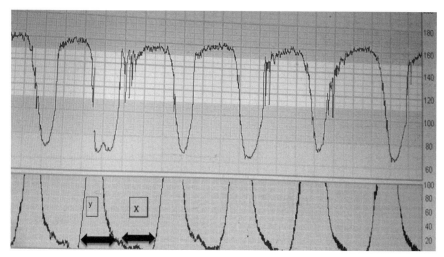

Figure 10.1 Intrapartum reoxygenation ratio ('x' divided by 'y').

- A more recent study by Bakker et al.[9] concluded that five or more contractions in 10 minutes during second stage of labour was associated with a higher incidence of neonatal acidaemia at birth when compared with contractions that were less frequent.
- A recent pilot study at St George's University Hospitals NHS Foundation Trust has shown that lower intrapartum reoxygenation ratio (<1) was associated with a 'pathological CTG' at the time of active second stage of labour (Figure 10.1). The average reoxygenation ratio in fetuses with Apgar scores <5 was lower (reoxygenation ratio <1) at both 1 and 10 minutes as compared to fetuses that had Apgar score >5.[10]

Key Features (Increased Uterine Activity)

An Acute Increase in Uterine Activity (e.g. Immediately after Increasing Oxytocin Infusion)

- Prolonged deceleration refers to a sudden drop in baseline heart rate (<110 bpm and usually <80 bpm). This may be short-lasting (up to 3 minutes) or prolonged (3–10 minutes).
- Baseline bradycardia refers to a baseline FHR <80 bpm persisting >10 minutes

Effects of Continuing Increase in Uterine Activity over Time

- Variable decelerations become more frequent, wider, and deeper – leading to an 'atypical' pattern.
- Disappearance of accelerations.
- Late decelerations (utero-placental insufficiency leading to acidosis).
- Baseline tachycardia (catecholamine surge), reduced baseline variability and stepladder pattern leading to bradycardia.

Key Pathophysiology behind Patterns Seen on the CTG Trace

- Physiologically, the frequent compression of uterine spiral arterioles without adequate relaxation time would result in diminished placental perfusion and impaired delivery of oxygen to the fetus, increasing the likelihood of fetal hypoxia and acidosis.
- Utero-placental insufficiency during labour results in the accumulation of carbon dioxide and hydrogen ions due to fetal metabolic acidosis that occurs secondary to anaerobic metabolism in the fetus.
- Increased carbon dioxide and hydrogen ion concentration coupled with decreased oxygen content of the fetal blood would stimulate the chemoreceptors, resulting in the activation of the parasympathetic component of the autonomic nervous system leading to a fall in the fetal heart.
- Chemoreceptor-mediated deceleration takes a longer time to recover because fresh oxygenated blood from the mother has to 'wash out' the accumulated acid and carbon dioxide after the cessation of a uterine contraction. Therefore, this results in a 'lag time' for FHR to recover back to its original baseline.
- As a fetus descends into maternal pelvis during the second stage of labour, it gets compressed leading to raised fetal intracranial pressure. Stimulation of the dura mater, which is richly supplied by the parasympathetic nervous system, leads to 'early' decelerations in the CTG trace.

Recommended Management

- If CTG abnormalities secondary to increased uterine activity are observed, oxytocin infusion should be immediately stopped (acute prolonged deceleration or loss of baseline FHR variability) or reduced (recurrent decelerations with stable baseline FHR and reassuring variability) based on the CTG abnormality.
- Abdominal examination to assess uterine activity (uterine tone, duration and frequency of contractions) and a vaginal examination to exclude an umbilical cord prolapse, rapid cervical dilatation, placental abruption and uterine scar dehiscence in case of previous caesarean sections should be performed. A fetal scalp electrode may be considered in the absence of 'acute intrapartum accidents'.
- Maternal blood pressure and pulse rate should be checked to exclude maternal hypotension.
- Intrauterine resuscitation (changing maternal position, administration of intravenous fluids – a 500 mL bolus of Hartmann solution) should be attempted.
- In cases of uterine hyperstimulation not resolving with initial measures, tocolysis (terbutaline 250 mcg subcutaneously) should be considered.
- Assess for recovery of fetal heart and a decrease in uterine activity, and, in the absence of acute intrapartum accidents, if the ongoing prolonged deceleration on the CTG trace does not recover by 9 minutes, then delivery should be expedited.

Pearls

- Early recognition of uterine hyperstimulation is crucial as poor utero-placental perfusion can result in impaired fetal perfusion and subsequent fetal compromise.
- Caution should be exercised while increasing the dose of oxytocin infusion because the uterine myometrium becomes progressively more sensitive to circulating oxytocin

due to the formation of oxytocin receptors on the fundus of the uterus with advancing labour.

Pitfalls

Pitfalls include failure to appreciate the effect of cumulative 'uterine activity' on the fetus and merely concentrating on the frequency of uterine contractions, as there is no clear information regarding cumulative uterine activity in most international guidelines.

- ACOG has defined tachysystole as over six contractions in a 10-minute window averaged >30 minutes. Based on fetal oxygenation studies, researchers have suggested to redefine this definition as over six in a 10-minute period with the possibility of decreased fetal oxygenation due to inadequate relaxation time between contractions. However, with the use of oxytocin, even three to four contractions may result in fetal hypoxic-ischaemic injury.
- Failure to take immediate measures to improve utero-placental circulation when evidence of fetal decompensation (loss of baseline variability or sudden prolonged deceleration) is observed. In such cases, in addition to stopping oxytocin infusion (or removal of prostaglandin pessary), tocolytics should be administered to improve utero-placental circulation.

Consequences of Mismanagement

- Mismanagement in second stage of labour can result in rapid development of fetal hypoxia, fetal decompensation and hypoxic injury leading to hypoxic-ischaemic encephalopathy.
- Failure to understand the pathophysiological changes behind features observed on the CTG trace may result in unnecessary surgical intervention with associated morbidity.
- Intrapartum fetal death or early neonatal death.
- Fetal hypoxic injury due to uterotonics is very difficult to defend from a medico-legal point of view as this is iatrogenic and preventable.

Exercises

1. A 25-year-old primigravida at 39 weeks of gestation presented with a history of spontaneous onset of labour. On vaginal examination, her cervix was 6 cm dilated with the presence of grade 2 meconium staining of the amniotic fluid.

   Four hours later, her labour was augmented with syntocinon (oxytocin) infusion as there was no progress of labour, and ongoing uterine contractions were deemed inadequate.

   Two hours after commencement of syntocinon infusion, uterine contractions were occurring 6 in 10 minutes each lasting 60 seconds on the CTG trace (Figure 10.2).

   a. What is your differential diagnosis?
   b. Is CTG monitoring indicated?
   c. What abnormalities will be noted on the CTG based on the differential diagnosis?
   d. What is your management?
   e. What will be noticed on the CTG trace if treatment is instituted?

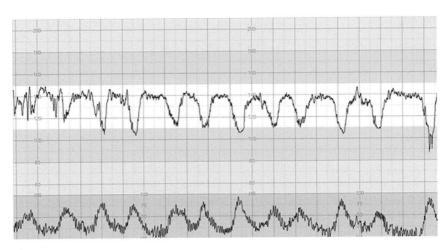

Figure 10.2

References

1. Rooth G, Huch A, Huch R. Guidelines for the use of fetal monitoring. *Int J Gynecol Obstet.* 1987; 25: 159–67.

2. Clinical Effectiveness Support Unit. The use of electronic fetal monitoring: The use of cardiotocography in intrapartum fetal surveillance. Evidence-based clinical guideline number 8. London: RCOG Press; 2001.

3. ACOG Technical Bulletin. Fetal heart rate patterns: monitoring, interpretation, and management. *Int J Gynecol Obstet.* 1995; 51: 65–74.

4. Uterine contraction monitoring. In: Freeman RK, Garite JY, Nageotte MP, eds. *Fetal heart monitoring*, 3rd ed. Philadelphia, PA: Lippincott Williams & Wilkins; 2003, pp. 54–62.

5. Fleisher A, Anyaegbunum AA, Schulman H, Farmakides G, Randolph G. Uterine and fetal umbilical artery velocimetry during normal labor. *Am J Obstet Gynecol.* 1987; 157: 40–3.

6. Brar HS, Platt LD, Devore GR, Horenstein J, Madearis AL. Qualitative assessment of maternal and fetal umbilical artery blood flow and resistance in laboring patients by Doppler velocimetry. *Am J Obstet Gynecol.* 1988; Apr; 158(4):952–6.

7. American College of Obstetricians and Gynaecologists, American Academy of Pediatrics. *Neonatal encephalopathy and cerebral palsy: Defining the pathogenesis and pathophysiology.* Washington, DC: ACOG and AAP; 2003.

8. McNamara H, Johnson N. The effect of uterine contractions on fetal oxygen saturation. *Br J Obstet Gynaecol.* 1995; 102: 644–7.

9. Bakker PCAM, Kurver PHJ, Kuik DJ, et al. Elevated uterine activity increases the risk of fetal acidosis at birth. *Am J Obstet Gynecol.* 2007; 196: 313e1–313.e6.

10. Muhammad S, Lowe V, Chandraharan E. Correlation between intrapartum re-oxygenation ratio and observed abnormalities on the CTG trace. *Singapore J Obstet Gynaec.* 2013; 44: 86.

Chapter

11

Intrapartum Monitoring of a Preterm Fetus

Ana Piñas Carrillo and Edwin Chandraharan

Key Facts

- The CTG patterns reflect the development and maturity of cardiac centres in the central nervous system and hence differ between preterm and term fetuses.
- Preterm fetuses, because of immaturity and low weight, are more likely to sustain intrapartum hypoxic injury. The physiological reserves are less than those in a well-grown term fetus, and in the presence of hypoxia, the compensatory response mounted by a preterm fetus is limited. The classical features observed on a CTG trace in the case of a term fetus may not be observed with the same amplitude in a preterm fetus. They have less capacity to release catecholamines due to smaller adrenal glands, and mild uterine contractions can easily cause variable decelerations due to a thinner umbilical cord with less Wharton jelly.
- The NICE guidelines, used in the UK, do not recommend intrapartum monitoring in preterm fetuses <37 weeks. In fact, none of the guidelines used worldwide (NICE, FIGO, ACOG) describe patterns of normality and CTG interpretation in fetuses <37 weeks of gestational age.
- Outcome between 24 and 28 weeks depends on maturity at birth and birth weight and not on the mode of delivery. Intrapartum monitoring of these fetuses can result on the misinterpretation of uncertain CTG patterns and unnecessary interventions that do not improve fetal outcome.
- Onset of preterm labour between 24 and 28 weeks is associated with infection in two-thirds of the cases. This presents an alternative pathway of fetal brain damage independent of hypoxia, and this inflammation-mediated neurological damage may be missed by the CTG trace.

Key Features on the CTG Trace

- Fetal baseline heart rate is higher at an average of 155 bpm at 24 weeks, and it decreases as pregnancy progresses, with fetuses having an average baseline heart rate of 140 bpm at term and 120 bpm at 41–42 weeks.
- The frequency and amplitude of accelerations are reduced before 30 weeks, frequently lasting for no longer than 10 seconds and with an increase of 10 bpm from baseline.
- The variability may also be reduced due to the immaturity of autonomic nervous system.

Handbook of CTG Interpretation: From Patterns to Physiology, ed. Edwin Chandraharan. Published by Cambridge University Press. © Cambridge University Press 2017.

- The presence of decelerations not related to contractions has also been described; typically, these are variable decelerations with low depth and duration. Up to 75 per cent of preterm fetuses may show intrapartum decelerations.

Key Pathophysiology behind Patterns Seen on the CTG Trace

- The baseline heart rate is maintained by the interaction of parasympathetic and sympathetic systems. Before 30 weeks, there is a predominance of the sympathetic system, and this results in an average higher baseline rate in preterm fetuses. As the parasympathetic system develops, it counteracts the activity of the sympathetic system, and the baseline rate decreases progressively from 30 weeks of gestation.
- Similarly, the baseline variability is maintained by the interaction between the two components of the autonomic nervous system. The lack of maturity of the parasympathetic system results in an apparent decrease in baseline variability, which is also influenced by the presence of baseline tachycardia secondary to unopposed sympathetic activity.
- The presence of decelerations not related to uterine contractions and the higher incidence of variable decelerations intrapartum (up to 75 per cent) in preterm fetuses can be explained by a decreased amount of amniotic fluid, reduced Wharton jelly in the cord and lack of maturity of the fetal myocardium and its glycogen stores.

Recommended Management

- CTG monitoring in fetuses <28 weeks is not recommended as no patterns of normality have been described. Monitoring these fetuses can result in unnecessary interventions (emergency caesarean section, instrumental delivery) that have been demonstrated not to improve the outcome of these extremely premature babies but have the potential to increase maternal morbidity.
- Beyond 32 weeks, survival rates vastly increase and hence fetal monitoring is recommended considering the special features that these fetuses show. Caution should be exercised between 28 and 32 weeks of gestation as no data is available on normality of CTG traces and how long abnormal features such as atypical or late decelerations could be allowed to persist prior to the onset of fetal decompensation.
- When interpreting CTG traces of fetuses between 28 and 36 + 6 weeks, it is essential to know its specific features and fetal physiological response. This can result in different management than when those same features are observed in a term fetus. For example, a preterm fetus at 28 weeks of gestation presenting with a baseline heart rate of 155 bpm in the absence of chorioamnionitis or maternal dehydration can be regarded as normal and will not require further intervention, whereas a fetus at 42 weeks of gestation presenting with the same baseline has to be closely monitored as it is likely to be an early sign of chorioamnionitis or an ongoing chronic hypoxia even in the absence of other clinical signs.
- If oxytocin augmentation is needed (i.e. due to severe sepsis) on a preterm fetus, the frequency of increase may need to be modified, as these fetuses are more likely to rapidly develop intrapartum hypoxia due to immaturity of the fetal compensatory response to stress.

- In the presence of tachycardia or reduced baseline variability, one should always exclude iatrogenic causes such as administration of drugs such as tocolytics (terbutaline), pethidine, magnesium sulphate and steroids.

Key Tips to Optimize Outcome

- *Fetuses 24–28 weeks of gestational age*: Continuous monitoring is not recommended. An isolated higher baseline FHR or reduced variability should not be considered a priori as abnormal and operative interventions are not indicated for such 'abnormal changes' on the CTG trace that merely reflect physiological immaturity of the autonomic nervous system. Remember that the physiological reserves to respond to hypoxia are not the same as in a term fetus, especially in the presence of chorioamnionitis.
- *Fetuses 28–32 weeks of gestational age*: Fetal monitoring may be considered as survival and neurological outcome significantly improves during this gestation. Fetal baseline heart rate and variability are often comparable to those of a term fetus, but accelerations can still be of a smaller magnitude. Always consider the clinical picture when interpreting the CTG trace (chorioamnionitis, drugs).
- *Fetuses 32–34 weeks*: The CTG trace can be classified according to the guidelines used on term fetuses. However, it is important to remember that the reserves in these fetuses are less than at term, and hence the ability to withstand a persistent hypoxic insult can be compromised (i.e. oxytocin augmentation).

Pitfalls

- Monitoring preterm fetuses between 24 and 28 weeks and acting on uncertain CTG patterns, leading to unnecessary interventions such as emergency caesarean section.
- Managing and interpreting CTG traces beyond 28 weeks as in a term fetus, unaware of the physiological reserves and the possibility of a growth-restricted fetus that has impaired response to hypoxic stress.
- Use of additional tests is not recommended for preterm fetuses. Fetal blood sampling has not been validated in this group, and fetal ECG (ST-Analyser) is unreliable because of changes in the myocardium composition (increased water content and less glycogen) and a smaller epicardial–endocardial interphase.

Consequences of Mismanagement

- Unnecessary operative deliveries
- Delivery of an extreme premature infant due to an overreaction to CTG patterns
- Stillbirth
- Neonatal death

Exercises

1. A 24-year-old primigravida presents at 28 weeks with reduced fetal movements. The CTG trace is shown in Figure 11.1.
   a. Classify the CTG applying the '8Cs' approach.
   b. What are the specific features different from those of a term fetus?
   c. What changes would you expect to see if you repeat the CTG in 4 weeks' time?
   d. How would you assess fetal well-being at this stage of pregnancy?

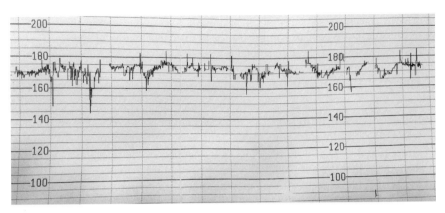

Figure 11.1

Further Reading

1. Afors K, Chandraharan E. Use of continuous electronic fetal monitoring in a preterm fetus: clinical dilemmas and recommendations for practice. *J Pregnancy.* 2011; 848794.

2. National Institute of Clinical Excellence. Intrapartum care: care of healthy women and their babies during childbirth. NICE clinical guideline CG190. December 2014.

3. Gibb D, Arulkumaran S. *Fetal Monitoring in Practice*. 3rd edn. Elsevier, 2008.

4. McDonnell S, Chandraharan E. The pathophysiology of CTGs and types of intrapartum hypoxia. *Curr. Women's Health Rev.* 2013; 9: 158–168.

5. Costeloe KL, Hennessy EM, Haider S, Stacey F, Marlow N, Draper ES. Short term outcomes after extreme preterm birth in England: comparison of two birth cohorts in 1995 and 2006 (the EPICure studies). *BMJ* 2012; 345: e7976.

Role of Chorioamnionitis and Infection

Jessica Moore and Edwin Chandraharan

Key Facts

- Chorioamnionitis is a significant cause of non-hypoxic fetal compromise.
- It may occur prior to the onset of labour or during the intrapartum period.
- Clinical chorioamnionitis is characterized by maternal pyrexia (≥38°C) and at least one of the following parameters: fetal tachycardia, maternal tachycardia, uterine tenderness, and/or offensive smelling liquor or purulent vaginal discharge.
- Meconium-stained liquor may also be a feature of chorioamnionitis.
- Once clinical chorioamnionitis is evident, it is likely that the infective process is well established in the fetoplacental unit.
- Histological chorioamnionitis is a presence of inflammatory cell infiltrates in the membranes of the placenta and in severe cases in the umbilical cord (funisitis).
- The presence of funisitis demonstrates the presence of a fetal systemic inflammatory response syndrome (FSIRS).
- The term subclinical chorioamnionitis is used when there are no overt signs of clinical chorioamnionitis but the placental histopathological examination reveals histological evidence of chorioamnionitis. This may manifest as preterm rupture of membranes or preterm labour or term pre-labour rupture of membranes (PROM).
- The term 'subclinical chorioamnionitis' may also refer to cases where intrauterine infection is suspected – such as maternal and fetal tachycardia with meconium-stained liquor. However, the criteria for clinical chorioamnionitis are not met. In addition, subclinical chorioamnionitis may present as preterm rupture of membranes or preterm labour.
- Adverse maternal outcomes with chorioamnionitis include postpartum haemorrhage from uterine atony, sepsis and postpartum endometritis.
- Adverse outcomes for the fetus include stillbirth, premature birth, neonatal infection, respiratory disease and brain injury and longer term sequelae such as learning difficulties and cerebral palsy.
- The presence of intrauterine infection is associated with a significantly increased risk of cerebral palsy. Clinical chorioamnionitis is associated with a fivefold increase in the risk of cerebral palsy, and histological chorioamnionitis an even higher risk of brain injury.
- Coexistence of intrauterine infection and hypoxia further increases the risk of cerebral palsy as compared to hypoxia alone (78- vs 5-fold as compared to background risk).

Handbook of CTG Interpretation: From Patterns to Physiology, ed. Edwin Chandraharan. Published by Cambridge University Press. © Cambridge University Press 2017.

- The relationship between severity of maternal disease in clinical chorioamnionitis and outcome for the fetus is unpredictable. In some cases, the mother may have significant signs of sepsis and yet the fetus may be born in good condition. Conversely, a mother may have no signs of clinical chorioamnionitis and yet the fetus may be born with significant systemic inflammation.
- It is vital to appreciate that chorioamnionitis is a fetal disease, and therefore, occurrence of maternal symptoms and signs may indicate an advanced fetal infection with poor neonatal outcome.
- Emerging scientific evidence suggests that inflammatory mediators per se can cause fetal neurological damage due to poor development of fetal blood–brain barrier without the presence of organisms within the amniotic cavity.

Risk factors and associations with chorioamnionitis include:

- Premature rupture of membranes and labour. It is likely that subclinical chorioamnionitis plays a role in the pathophysiology of premature rupture of membranes. However, once this occurs, there is an increased risk of clinical chorioamnionitis due to ascending infection.
- Prolonged rupture of membranes.
- Group B streptococcal colonization in the mother.

Key Pathophysiology of Infection and CTG

- The understanding of CTG changes in the presence of fetal infection is poor. Chorioamnionitis may lead to FSIRS.
- It is possible that fetal inflammatory response may cause neurological injury through different mechanisms to those caused by hypoxia although there may be common synergetic pathways. Although it is possible that with infection there is no protective upregulation of anti-inflammatory cytokines which occurs in fetal hypoxic ischaemia.
- The possible mechanisms of fetal brain injury include a reduction in oxygen transfer across inflamed fetal membranes or a reduction in fetal cardiac output secondary to myocardial dysfunction causing a reduction in cerebral blood flow.
- Severe fetal infection may result in a metabolic acidosis although often the cord pH may be normal despite the fetus being born in poor condition.
- Fetal infection in the presence of ongoing hypoxic stress will result in a worse outcome for the fetus. This is because inflammatory mediators lower the threshold at which hypoxia can cause fetal neurological damage.

Key Features on the CTG Trace

- It must be remembered that CTG monitoring is a test for fetal hypoxia and that the role of CTG in chorioamnionitis is less clear.
- There is a lack of evidence that specific features on the CTG trace can identify cases of clinical or subclinical chorioamnionitis. However, understanding the pathophysiology of hypoxia and FSIRS may help in recognizing ongoing clinical or subclinical chorioamnionitis based on the features observed on the CTG trace.

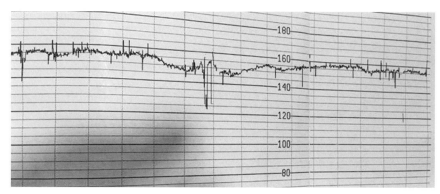

Figure 12.1 CTG features associated with chorioamnionitis at term. Note the absence of cycling and accelerations with the baseline FHR at or above the upper limit of normal.

- It is probably important to consider the features of a term CTG separately to those in a preterm CTG.
- Studies that have looked at the role of CTG in the identification of systemic fetal infection have often applied the definitions used for hypoxia, and it is possible that intra-amniotic infection exerts an effect on the fetus through different pathways. This may explain why many of the studies evaluating the CTG in fetal infection have not been conclusive.
- CTG features seen in the presence of intrauterine infection include fetal tachycardia, reduced variability, lack of accelerations, presence of decelerations and lack of cycling (Figure 12.1), but none of these features have been seen consistently.
- 'Saltatory pattern' (variability >25 bpm) may be seen in maternal pyrexia due to the dysregulation of fetal thermoregulatory centre.
- One study estimated that fetal tachycardia at term was associated with an increased risk of systemic fetal inflammation of 9 times the odds of a term fetus with no tachycardia. There is also evidence that fetal tachycardia increases the incidence of cerebral palsy.
- If fetal tachycardia and reduced variability are seen without preceding or on-going decelerations, then consideration should be given to infection as the primary cause. This is because fetal tachycardia will be almost always preceded by decelerations in cases of intrapartum hypoxia.
- It is important to compare FHR with any previously recorded FHR as a significant rise in FHR should prompt the question of infection.
- Ongoing baseline fetal tachycardia on admission or in early labour in a term fetus may be suggestive of underlying subclinical chorioamnionitis. This should prompt a clinician to look for other signs of maternal inflammatory response. In the absence of a diagnosis of clinical chorioamnionitis, the patient should be observed closely for evolving signs (maternal tachycardia, maternal pyrexia, meconium staining of amniotic fluid or an offensive vaginal discharge).
- Other causes of fetal tachycardia such as maternal hypotension, dehydration, chronic hypoxia and medications (e.g. salbutamol) should be excluded.

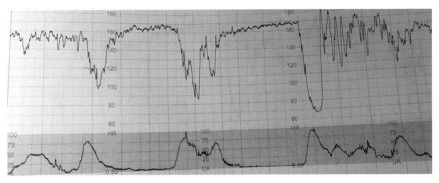

Figure 12.2. Onset of atypical variable decelerations on the background of fetal tachycardia secondary to clinical or subclinical chorioamnionitis. Such a combination of hypoxia and infection can potentiate fetal neurological injury.

Recommended Management

- If clinical chorioamnionitis is diagnosed, then a full septic screening of the mother should be undertaken along with the administration of broad-spectrum intravenous antibiotics and antipyretics.
- One should not rely on the CTG as a test of fetal well-being when clinical chorioamnionitis is present. However, evidence of coexisting intrapartum hypoxia (i.e. presence of repetitive atypical variable or late decelerations) is a bad prognostic indicator.
- Consider expediting delivery. It is difficult to give exact timing for when delivery should occur. However, if subclinical chorioamnionitis is suspected, care should be taken to avoid further hypoxic stress on the fetus due to the synergistic damaging effect of hypoxia and infection on the fetal brain.
- If a diagnosis of clinical chorioamnionitis is made prior to delivery, consideration should be given to delivery by caesarean section to avoid any additional hypoxic stress from labour (e.g. primigravida with cervical dilatation <6 cm, or if there is evidence of failure to progress requiring oxytocin augmentation).
- Avoidance of additional hypoxic stress (e.g. repetitive cord compression or increased uterine activity leading to reduced utero-placental oxygenation) is paramount (Figure 12.2). This means oxytocin should be used with great caution, and it is prudent to avoid a prolonged labour or a complicated delivery.
- If labour is progressing quickly and vaginal delivery is anticipated within the next 3–4 hours, it is appropriate to continue with labour if the CTG trace is entirely normal suggestive of no ongoing hypoxic stress.
- Partogram should be carefully scrutinized to monitor the progress in labour closely as well as any signs of deterioration in the condition of mother or fetus.
- Consider the mode of delivery. There is a lack of evidence that caesarean section at the time of diagnosis of clinical chorioamnionitis will improve the neonatal outcome. However, there is a significant association between duration of chorioamnionitis and 5-minute Apgar score <3 and mechanical ventilation within 24 hours.
- Ensure a neonatologist is present at delivery.

- Take umbilical cord gases in confirmed or suspected clinical chorioamnionitis.
- The placenta should have a swab taken for microscopy and culture and the placenta should be sent for histopathological examination.

Key Tips to Optimize Outcome

- Consider infection as a cause for fetal tachycardia especially in the absence of decelerations and look for other signs to confirm this.
- Consider infection as a cause of loss of cycling in the CTG suggestive of depression of the central nervous system.
- Consider delivery by caesarean section especially if vaginal delivery is not imminent (i.e. if cervix <6 cm in a primigravida, or if there is evidence of failure to progress).
- Remember to look at the whole clinical picture when managing a labour with suspected infection.
- Remember that infection will cause morbidity and mortality in mother and fetus. The correlation between severity of maternal disease and neonatal outcome is not clear.
- Avoid coexisting intrapartum hypoxia as it will have a synergistic effect with infection.
- Consider other causes of maternal pyrexia such as use of epidural medications and drugs. However, be aware that pyrexia of any cause is associated with an increased incidence of neonatal seizures.
- Meconium may be associated with ongoing clinical and subclinical chorioamnionitis as it may indicate ongoing fetal stress secondary to infection. Conversely, meconium may reduce the antibacterial activity of the amniotic fluid and may predispose to chorioamnionitis. Therefore, presence of meconium with ongoing fetal tachycardia is an ominous sign and delivery should be expedited.

Pitfalls

- A failure to consider infection as a cause of abnormal CTG which does not fit into a hypoxic pattern (i.e. absence of repetitive decelerations).
- A failure to appreciate that even mild hypoxia in the context of clinical chorioamnionitis will have worse prognosis.
- Failure to incorporate the whole clinical picture, e.g., primparous, early labour, thick meconium, pyrexia and fetal tachycardia may lead to poor outcomes and these cases are likely to benefit from an early delivery by a caesarean section.
- Performing additional tests of fetal well-being such as fetal scalp blood sampling (FBS), fetal scalp lactate or fetal ECG (ST-Analyser). None of these tests designed to diagnose intrapartum hypoxia are reliable in fetal infection.

Consequences of Mismanagement

- Intrapartum fetal death
- Early neonatal death
- Severe neonatal sepsis
- Long-term sequelae such as learning difficulties and cerebral palsy

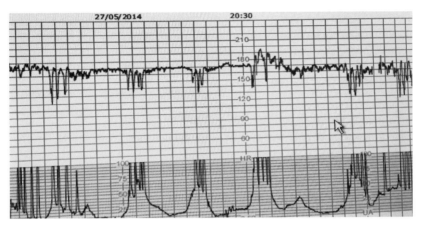

Figure 12.3

Exercises

1. A primigravida was admitted for induction of labour at 41 weeks + 3 days of gestation. She had no antenatal risk factors. CTG trace was commenced (Figure 12.3).
   a. How would you classify the CTG trace?
   b. What is your management plan?

   A plan was made for expectant management and the maternal pulse rate was noted to be 108 bpm.

   c. What is the likely diagnosis?
   d. What is your management plan?
   f. What are the signs and symptoms you would be anticipating in this case?

   A plan was made to continue with labour. Three hours later, maternal temperature was recorded as 38.2°C. Paracetamol and intravenous antibiotics were administered. Six hours later, cervix was found to be 4 cm dilated and artificial rupture of membranes was carried out and meconium staining of amniotic fluid was noted.

   g. What is your diagnosis?
   h. What is your management plan and why?

Further Reading

1. Aina-Mumuney AJ, Althaus JE, Henderson JL, et al. Intrapartum electronic fetal monitoring and the identification of systemic fetal inflammation. *J Reprod Med.* 2007; 52: 762–768.

2. Badawi N, Kurinczuk JJ, Keogh JM, et al. Intrapartum risk factors for newborn encephalopathy: the Western Australian

case-control study. *BMJ.* 1998; 317: 1554–1558.

3. Peebles DM, Wyatt JS. Synergy between antenatal exposure to infection and intrapartum events in causation of perinatal brain injury at term. *BJOG.* 2002; 109: 737–739.

4. Rouse JR, Landon M, Leveno KJ. The maternal-fetal units caesarean registry: chorioamnionitis at term and its duration–relationship outcomes. *Am J Obstet Gynaecol.* 2004; 191: 211–2116.

5. Sameshima H, Ikenoue T, Ikeda T, et al. Association of non-reassuring fetal heart rate patterns and subsequent cerebral palsy in pregnancies with intrauterine bacterial infection. *Am J Perinatol.* 2005; 22: 181–187.

6. Tita A, Andrews W. Diagnosis and management of clinical chorioamnionitis. *Clin Perinatol.* 2010; 37: 339–354.

7. Ugwumadu A. Infection and fetal neurological injury. *Curr Opin Obstet Gynaecol.* 2006; 18: 106–111.

8. Wu YW, Escobar GJ, Grether JK. Chorioamnionitis and cerebral palsy in term and near term infants. *JAMA.* 2003; 290: 2677–2684.

Chapter 3

Meconium

Why Is It Harmful?

Nirmala Chandrasekaran and Leonie Penna

Key Facts

Causes of meconium

Physiological: As the fetal gut reaches maturity, peristaltic contractions of the bowel occur spontaneously as part of normal development. Forty-four per cent of fetuses beyond 42 weeks of gestation will have passed meconium. The majority of cases of meconium-stained amniotic fluid (MSAF) at term are physiological. Physiological meconium is always light as there should be a normal volume of amniotic fluid, and as it is rare for meconium to be passed by the fetus before 37 weeks, gestation will usually be beyond 37 weeks with even greater reassurance offered by postterm gestations. There should be no risk factors for placental insufficiency, intrapartum hypoxia or infection in order to consider meconium as physiological. The parasympathetic nervous system increases overall gut motility, and thus meconium can be passed during labour as a result of head compression via a vagally mediated response. This response is uncommon during the first stage of labour and is most commonly seen in the passage of meconium during the late second stage in healthy infants born with no evidence of infection or acidosis.

Fetal hypoxia: Reduction in the amount of oxygen available to a fetus in labour results in an adrenergic response with a rising fetal heart rate (FHR) and redistribution of blood to essential organs with a reduction in blood flow to nonessential organs including the bowel. This and a direct vagal effect can result in peristaltic bowel contractions and relaxation of the anal sphincter resulting in the passage of meconium. This effect is most commonly seen in a gradually developing hypoxia and may not occur in chronic long-standing hypoxia or in acute severe hypoxia (such as massive abruption).

Maternal obstetric cholestasis: MSAF is more common in woman with a diagnosis of obstetric cholestasis especially where bile acids are >40 micromoles per litre with rates of 25 per cent reported in term and 18 per cent in preterm labour.

Fetal bowel abnormality: Gastroschisis increases the likelihood of MSAF during labour (including preterm). The reason for this effect is not certain but is possibly due to the direct contact of the bowel with the amniotic fluid stimulating peristaltic contractions.

Listeriosis: Fetal listeria infection is reported to cause MSAF in preterm labour but is very rare and unlikely to be the cause of MSAF. Maternal blood cultures should be taken for listeria, but other infective pathologies or hypoxia are more common and should be considered.

Handbook of CTG Interpretation: From Patterns to Physiology, ed. Edwin Chandraharan. Published by Cambridge University Press. © Cambridge University Press 2017.

Fetal infection: Meconium increases the risk of chorioamnionitis as it inhibits neutrophil phagocytosis and as a result enhances bacterial growth.

Recommended Management

- CTG monitoring must always be considered in labours complicated by meconium-stained liquor because of its association with hypoxia and infection. However, the fact that most meconium is physiological has resulted in conflicts regarding the level of intervention appropriate in the low-risk pregnancy.

- The woman should be advised that in the majority of cases meconium represents a physiological response in the maturing fetus but that in a small number of cases it may be an indicator of a fetal problem and that it is important to detect any falling oxygen levels as this may result in fetuses gasping with the effect of meconium entering their lungs causing meconium aspiration syndrome (MAS). The importance of fetal monitoring in identifying a fetus that is becoming stressed by labour should be explained with reassurance that this monitoring is effective.

- For thin meconium in gestations >37 weeks with no risk factors for placental insufficiency or infection, continuous electronic fetal monitoring (CEFM) is not deemed mandatory by some national guidelines. However, intermittent auscultation (IA) and maternal observations for signs of sepsis must be performed to the highest standard with immediate conversion to CEFM if any new risk factor or pyrexia develops or there are concerns about the quality or findings of IA (e.g. a progressive rise in baseline FHR).

- In any type of meconium with any risk factor for infection or development of intrauterine hypoxia, CEFM should be recommended and commenced for the duration of labour. CEFM should also be recommended for thin MSAF in women with previous clear liquor who develop meconium as a new finding or if labour becomes prolonged.

- If fetal heart monitoring is normal, then no specific action is required regardless of the type of meconium or the presence of signs of infection. With thick meconium and possible infection, a careful review of labour progress is prudent, with delivery considered if the interval until spontaneous delivery is likely to take many hours.

- In order to ensure that management is optimized, it is important to consider the underlying pathophysiology that may be indicated by the trace. Table 13.1 summarizes a suggested plan of management for CEFM in the presence of meconium.

- Thin meconium does not alter the way CEFM should be interpreted, as in the majority of cases it will be of physiological aetiology. The possibility of infection should be considered and if there is any possibility of chorioamnionitis, then monitoring should be managed as if meconium were heavy.

- CEFM showing a suspicious type pattern usually indicates a fetus that is under stress, either a mechanical one (cord compression decelerations) or a possible infection (an uncomplicated tachycardia) with risk of developing hypoxia. Urgent clinical review with interventions to improve the fetal condition is implemented (intravenous fluids and optimization of maternal position). The interplay of sepsis, meconium and hypoxia must be considered along with the likelihood that fetal stress can be effectively reduced and the expected interval until spontaneous delivery. Care must be individualized, but a decision to recommend immediate delivery by C-section should be considered in cases with abnormal monitoring and possible sepsis where spontaneous delivery (or

Table 13.1 Suggested plan of management for CEFM in the presence of meconium

	Quantification of meconium			
	Light		Heavy	
	Is there possible infection (fetal tachycardia, maternal tachycardia or maternal pyrexia?			
	No	Yes	No	Yes
CTG assessment				
Normal CTG	Offer IA if low risk or recommend CEFM if risk factors	Recommend CEFM, intravenous antibiotics, careful observation of CTG	Recommend CEFM and careful surveillance for signs of infection	CEFM, intravenous antibiotics, consider probability and timing of spontaneous delivery
Suspicious CTG	Recommend CEFM, intrauterine resuscitation measures and observe carefully	Recommend CEFM, intravenous antibiotics	Recommend CEFM, reconsider risk of infection and delivery if vaginal birth is not imminent	CEFM, intravenous antibiotics, assisted delivery unless spontaneous delivery imminent
Abnormal CTG	Recommend CEFM, intrauterine resuscitation	Recommend CEFM, intravenous antibiotics delivery if vaginal delivery is not imminent	Recommend CEFM, or delivery depending on the probability of spontaneous delivery, reconsider risk of infection	CEFM, intravenous antibiotics, urgent assisted delivery by C-section or assisted vaginal delivery unless delivery immediately imminent

Caution: Additional tests of fetal well-being such as fetal scalp blood sampling (FBS) and fetal ECG (ST-Analyser) are not useful in predicting MAS. In addition, scientific evidence suggests that FBS can provide a false-positive result as meconium contains bile acids which alter the pH of fetal scalp sample due to contamination.

assisted vaginal delivery) is not imminent. If the decision is made to continue, then continuous FHR monitoring should be performed as fetal hypoxia may develop faster in the presence of meconium. Where possible, clinical decisions should be made to avoid deterioration of such a trace to become pathological. A true reduction in baseline variability (<5 bpm) or development of saltatory pattern on a previously 'suspicious' CTG trace would be particularly ominous in the circumstance and should be managed without delay as a pathological trace.

- CEFM showing a pathological type pattern with a much greater risk that the fetus has significant hypoxia (usually a complicated baseline tachycardia but occasionally reduced variability on an admission CTG of a woman in labour with thick meconium) requires delivery to be expedited by C-section or assisted vaginal delivery. A senior clinician should be involved in the decision-making process with clear documentation of the thinking behind the decision. It is important to appreciate that additional tests of fetal well-being such as FBS and fetal ECG (ST-Analyser or STAN) are not useful in predicting MAS. FBS may give a false-positive result as the presence of bile acids in meconium may reduce the pH of scalp blood sample.
- Increased baseline FHR and presence of repeated atypical or prolonged decelerations indicative of ongoing hypoxia may increase the likelihood of MAS.

- In cases of MSAF with a gestation <37 weeks, immediate CEFM and urgent review by a senior obstetrician to formulate a plan for delivery are recommended. Any abnormality in FHR monitoring or evidence of sepsis requires consideration of expediting delivery by C-section unless vaginal delivery is imminent. FBS is not recommended as a lack of fetal reserve in the premature fetus and an increased likelihood of infection in combination with meconium is a situation when the rate of development of hypoxia is unpredictable.

Common Pitfalls

- Failure to recommend monitoring in women with risk factors for hypoxia or infection presenting with MSAF.
- UK guidelines for the interpretation of CEFM do not make specific recommendation about how interpretation should be altered by the finding of significant meconium.
- Not considering infection risks when formulating a management plan for a labour complicated by meconium.
- Delaying delivery in the presence of developing hypoxia with the risk of fetal gasping in utero.

Consequences of Meconium

- Cerebral palsy is twice as common in term infants with MSAF than in infants with clear fluid. In preterm labour, it is an even higher risk factor for future neurologic disorder with one study showing that 41 per cent of premature infants born with MSAF develop cerebral palsy, compared to 10 per cent of preterm infants with clear amniotic fluid.
- Neonatal MAS is the result of aspiration of acidic meconium causing chemical pneumonitis with cytokine activation and development of persistent pulmonary hypertension. Any developing hypoxia increases the risk of fetal gasping in utero and this increases the risk of MAS.

Further Reading

Hofmeyr GJ, Xu H, Eke AC. Amnioinfusion for meconium-stained liquor in labour. *Cochrane Database Syst Rev.* 2014; 1.

National Institute for Health and Care Excellence. Intrapartum care: care of healthy women and their babies during childbirth. Clinical guideline 55. 2007.

National Institute for Health and Care Excellence. Intrapartum care: care of healthy women and their babies during childbirth. Clinical guideline 109. 2014.

Siriwachirachai T, Sangkomkamhang US, Lumbiganon P, Laopaiboon M. Antibiotics for meconium stained amniotic fluid in labour for preventing maternal and neonatal infection. *Cochrane Database Syst Rev.* 2014; 11.

Intrapartum Bleeding

Edwin Chandraharan

Key Facts

- Intrapartum vaginal bleeding may be benign – damage to maternal veins during cervical dilatation, or rupture of membranes – or may indicate serious underlying pathology.
- Serious causes include rupture of fetal blood vessels traversing the membranes below the presenting part (vasa previa), placental abruption, bleeding from a low-lying placenta (placenta previa), uterine rupture or, rarely, bleeding from local lesions such as polyps, tumours, or genital tract trauma.

Key Features on the CTG Trace

- Maternal causes of intrapartum bleeding often do not cause any change on the CTG trace, unless it is very severe and is accompanied by maternal hypotension (e.g. placenta previa). If this is a case, an acute prolonged deceleration will be noted on the CTG trace.
- Bleeding from vasa previa or a sudden fetomaternal haemorrhage may result in an 'atypical sinusoidal pattern' also called 'Poole shark teeth pattern' (Figure 14.1).
- Premature separation of placenta may result in recurrent 'late decelerations' (Figure 14.2) in early stages but may result in an acute prolonged deceleration culminating in a terminal bradycardia (see Chapter 2). A total loss of baseline fetal heart rate (FHR) variability may also be noted (Figure 14.2).
- Uterine rupture may present with recurrent variable or late decelerations or as an acute prolonged deceleration (see Chapter 15).

Key Pathophysiology behind Patterns Seen on the CTG Trace

- Atypical sinusoidal pattern is believed to occur secondary to acute fetal hypotension and resultant acute hypoxia to the central nervous system that causes instability of the autonomic nervous system (sympathetic and parasympathetic).
- Recurrent 'late decelerations' (Figure 14.2) in early stages of abruption is secondary to utero-placental insufficiency and metabolic acidosis resulting in the stimulation of chemoreceptors. Acute prolonged deceleration culminating in a terminal bradycardia is

Handbook of CTG Interpretation: From Patterns to Physiology, ed. Edwin Chandraharan. Published by Cambridge University Press. © Cambridge University Press 2017.

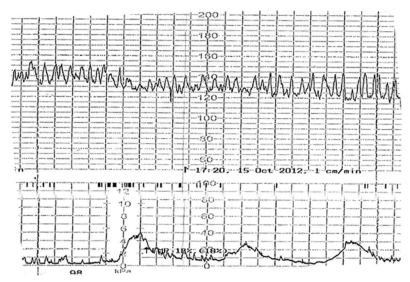

Figure 14.1

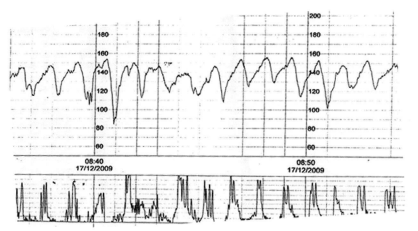

Figure 14.2. Note the total loss of baseline fetal heart rate variability within the first 3 minutes of a prolonged deceleration

secondary to myocardial decompensation resulting from hypoxia and acidosis due to a total disruption of the fetal oxygen supply (see Chapter 2). A sudden reduction in fetal blood volume and resultant lack of oxygen supply to the brain results in a total loss of baseline FHR variability (Figure 14.2).

- Recurrent variable decelerations may occur secondary to prolapsed umbilical cord through the ruptured uterine scar, and late decelerations occur secondary to progressive placental separation leading to progressive fetal hypoxia and acidosis and resultant 'chemoreceptor stimulation' (Figure 14.3). An acute prolonged deceleration may occur secondary to expulsion of the fetus into the peritoneal cavity that results in a total separation of the placenta (see Chapter 15).

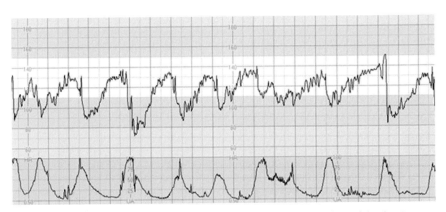

Figure 14.3 Note the presence of decelerations prior to the onset of the prolonged deceleration.

Recommended Management

- In cases of fetomaternal haemorrhage or placental abruption presenting with CTG changes suggestive of ongoing fetal hypoxia or hypotension, urgent delivery should be accomplished by the quickest and safest approach. If the cervix is fully dilated with presenting part at or below the ischial spines, an immediate operative vaginal delivery is recommended. If this is not possible, then an immediate ('grade 1') caesarean section should be performed.
- The neonatal team should be informed as the neonate may be hypoxic and hypotensive at birth requiring intensive neonatal resuscitation as well as intravenous fluids and blood transfusion to correct ongoing hypovolaemia.
- In cases of severe abruption with maternal hypotension and coagulopathy, maternal resuscitation should take priority while making preparations for urgent delivery. Maternal oxygen administration used in cases of maternal collapse may also have a beneficial effect on the fetus.

Key Tips to Optimize Outcome

- Recognize atypical sinusoidal pattern and/or acute prolonged deceleration when there is ongoing fetomaternal bleeding secondary to a vasa previa (Figure 14.3) or a concealed abruption.
- Remember that baseline FHR variability will be rapidly reduced within first 3 minutes of a prolonged deceleration due to ongoing fetal hypotension and resultant sudden reduction in fetal cerebral blood flow.
- Seek immediate senior obstetric and midwifery input and ensure effective multidisciplinary communication and team working to accomplish immediate delivery.

Pitfalls

- '3, 6, 9, 12, 15' rule for a prolonged deceleration is not applicable in this case.
- Persists with traumatic operative vaginal delivery despite ongoing features on the CTG suggestive of acute hypoxia.

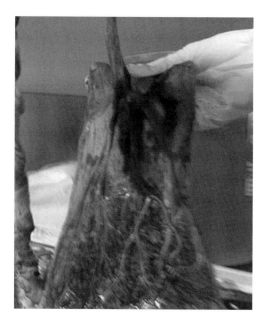

Figure 14.4 Note the ruptured vasa praevia in a case with an atypical sinusoidal pattern with a 'jagged edge' resembling 'Poole Shark Teeth'.

- Attempting additional tests of fetal well-being such as fetal ECG (STAN), fetal scalp pH or lactate when there is clear evidence of hypoxia to the central organs on the CTG trace.

Consequences of Mismanagement
- Intrapartum fetal death
- Early neonatal death
- Severe hypoxic ischaemic encephalopathy (HIE)
- Long-term fetal neurological sequelae secondary to delayed treatment of hypotension

Exercise
1. A 36-year-old primigravida presented with a history of painless vaginal bleeding with reduced fetal movements at 40 weeks of gestation. On examination, the abdomen was soft and nontender and FHR was 160 bpm. On speculum examination, fresh vaginal bleeding was noted.
   a. What is your differential diagnosis?
   b. Is CTG monitoring indicated?
   c. What abnormalities on the CTG would be expected based on your differential diagnosis?
   d. CTG was commenced and the following features were noted (Figure 14.5). What is your diagnosis?
   e. What is your management?

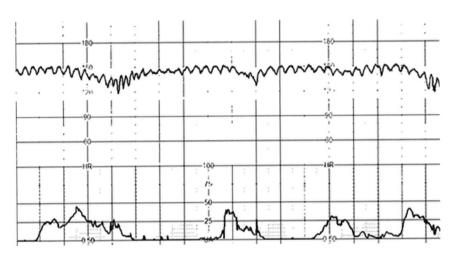

Figure 14.5

Further Reading

1. Chandraharan E, Arulkumaran S. Prevention of birth asphyxia: responding appropriately to cardiotocograph (CTG) traces. *Best Pract Res Clin Obstet Gynaecol.* 2007; 21(4): 609–24.

2. Gibb D, Arulkumaran S (Eds). *Fetal monitoring in practice.* Elsevier. 2008.

3. Yanamandra N, Chandraharan E. Saltatory and sinusoidal fetal heart rate patterns and significance of FHR 'overshoots'. *Curr. Women's Health Revs.* 2013; 9: 175–82.

4. Jensen A, Hanson MA. Circulatory responses to acute asphyxia in intact and chemodenervated fetal sheep near term. *Reprod Fertil Dev.* 1995; 7: 1351–9.

5. Graca LM, Cardoso CG, Calhaz-Jorge C. An approach to interpretation and classification of sinusoidal fetal heart rate patterns. *Eur J Obstet Gynecol Reprod Biol.* 1988; 27: 203–12.

Chapter

15

Labour with a Uterine Scar
The Role of CTG

Ana Piñas Carrillo and Edwin Chandraharan

Key Facts

- Uterine scar dehiscence refers to the disruption of uterine myometrium but with an intact serosa (peritoneal covering), whereas uterine rupture refers to the total disruption of the entire uterine wall, including the serosa.
- The increasing rate of caesarean sections in modern obstetric practice is responsible for the rise in the number of women labouring with a previous uterine scar.
- Labour in the presence of a uterine scar has a risk of uterine rupture of 0.5 per cent in spontaneous labour, 0.8 per cent with the use of oxytocin for augmentation of labour and 2.4 per cent with the use of prostaglandins for induction of labour.
- The dehiscence/rupture of the uterus compromises the placental circulation, and this results in fetal heart rate (FHR) changes, frequently one of the first signs of uterine rupture. Continuous intrapartum fetal monitoring is essential in order to diagnose the onset of FHR abnormalities so as to institute timely delivery to avoid maternal and fetal complications.
- The classical signs of uterine rupture such as vaginal bleeding, scar or abdominal pain, receding presenting part, changes in the shape of the uterus and palpation of fetal parts are not always present and often unreliable.

Key Features on the CTG Trace

- The CTG features observed depend on the type of dehiscence/rupture.
- Uterine rupture can result in a prolonged deceleration lasting >3 minutes. The specific features that should elicit a high index of suspicion of uterine rupture include a total loss of variability within the first 3 minutes of deceleration, FHR dropping >60 bpm from the initial baseline and/or baseline FHR dropping <80 bpm. This may be associated with a sustained contraction (uterine hypertonus) or a sudden cessation of uterine activity recorded on the 'toco' component of the CTG.
- Repetitive variable or late decelerations and reduced variability may be observed preceding a final prolonged deceleration.
- Uterine rupture is frequently preceded by tachysystole (presence of more than five contractions in 10 minutes without CTG changes) or hyperstimulation (increased frequency, duration or tone of uterine contractions associated with changes on the CTG trace).

Handbook of CTG Interpretation: From Patterns to Physiology, ed. Edwin Chandraharan. Published by Cambridge University Press. © Cambridge University Press 2017.

Key Pathophysiology behind Patterns Seen on the CTG Trace

- Recurrent variable decelerations may occur secondary to prolapsed loop of umbilical cord through the ruptured uterine scar into the peritoneal cavity, and its resultant compression and late decelerations occur secondary to progressive placental separation leading to progressive fetal hypoxia and acidosis and resultant 'chemoreceptor stimulation'.
- An acute prolonged deceleration may occur secondary to the expulsion of the fetus into the peritoneal cavity that results in a total separation of the placenta. If this persists for >10 minutes, it is termed terminal bradycardia.

Recommended Management

- In cases of uterine rupture presenting with acute hypoxia shown on the CTG trace by a prolonged deceleration, immediate laparotomy to avoid fetal hypoxic-ischaemic injury and delivery within 10–15 minutes (category 1 caesarean section) is indicated in this situation. If delivery is imminent, one should consider immediate operative vaginal delivery followed by a laparotomy for repair to avoid fetal hypoxic ischaemic injury.
- The neonatal team should be informed of the suspicion of uterine rupture as it is likely that the fetus will be born in poor condition and would need intensive neonatal resuscitation, especially in cases of complete uterine rupture when the fetus is found extruded in the abdominal cavity.
- In women labouring with a previous uterine scar, the presence of repetitive variable and late decelerations and reduced variability should arouse a high index of suspicion of uterine dehiscence/rupture, and this needs to be excluded before continuing with labour.
- The use of transabdominal ultrasound scan to detect free fluid within the abdominal cavity or disruption of the myometrium with bulging membranes may be useful in cases where there is a strong clinical suspicion but with no classical symptoms and signs of uterine rupture and when the changes observed on the CTG are less marked or just 'suspicious'.
- In the presence of uterine tachysystole in a patient with a previous uterine scar, clinicians should consider tocolysis even in the absence of FHR changes to avoid the risk of uterine rupture.

Key Tips to Optimize Outcome

- Baseline FHR variability will be rapidly reduced within the first 3 minutes of a prolonged deceleration due to ongoing fetal hypotension and resultant sudden reduction in fetal cerebral blood flow.
- Seek immediate senior obstetric and midwifery input and ensure effective multidisciplinary communication and team working to accomplish immediate delivery.
- If the CTG trace before the prolonged deceleration was normal, scientific evidence suggests that if the delivery is accomplished within 18 minutes, fetal neurological injury is unlikely. However, if there are already ongoing decelerations prior to

the onset of acute prolonged deceleration, fetal neurological injury may ensue after 10 minutes.

Pitfalls

- '3, 6, 9, 12, 15' rule for a prolonged deceleration is not applicable in this case. Immediate delivery is indicated.
- Relying on vaginal bleeding or abdominal pain to diagnose uterine rupture in the presence of a suspicious trace should be avoided. These symptoms are commonly absent; looking at the clinical picture (use of oxytocin and/or prostaglandins, hyperstimulation, sustained contraction) together with the CTG features should arouse a suspicion of uterine rupture/dehiscence.
- Attempting additional tests of fetal well-being such as fetal ECG (STAN), fetal scalp pH or lactate when there is clear evidence of hypoxia to the central organs on the CTG trace should be avoided as it would merely delay delivery and worsen maternal and fetal complications.

Consequences of Mismanagement

- Intrapartum fetal death
- Early neonatal death
- Severe hypoxic ischaemic encephalopathy
- Long-term fetal neurological sequelae secondary to delayed treatment of hypotension
- Maternal collapse, need for multiple blood transfusion and, rarely, maternal death

Exercise

1. A 36-year-old gravida 2 para 1 with a previous caesarean section for failure to progress in labour was admitted with spontaneous onset of labour. Cervix was 6 cm dilated and the presenting part was at 0 station and the CTG trace was classified as normal. Oxytocin was commenced at 23:00 hours for failure to progress in labour as her cervix had remained 6 cm 2 hours after artificial rupture of membranes.
   a. Classify the CTG trace (using the '8C' format).
   b. What are effects of oxytocin on myometrial contractions and what changes would you observe on the CTG trace?
   c. Consider the CTG trace from 02:58 hours.
      1. What is the type of hypoxia?
      2. What are the differential diagnoses?
      3. What immediate actions would you take?
   d. What is the likelihood of the observed CTG change to return back to normal in this case?
   e. What would you expect to see in the umbilical cord gases if delivery was accomplished within 20 minutes of the onset of this acute, prolonged decelerations?

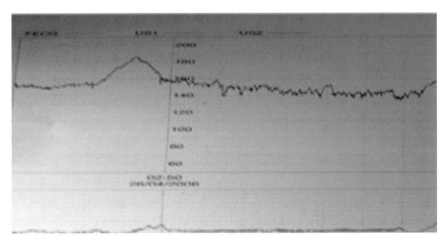

Figure 15.1

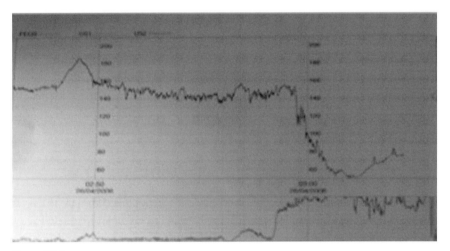

Figure 15.2

Further Reading

1. Gibb D, Arulkumaran S. *Fetal Monitoring in Practice*. 3rd edn. Elsevier, 2008.

2. Chandraharan E, Arulkumaran S. *Obstetric and Intrapartum Emergencies. A Practical Guide to Management*. Cambridge, 2012.

3. Chandraharan E. Rational approach to electronic fetal monitoring during labour in 'all' resource settings. *Sri Lanka J Obstet Gynaecol*. 2010; 32: 77–84.

4. McDonnell S, Chandraharan E. The pathophysiology of CTGs and types of intrapartum hypoxia. *Curr Women's Health Revs*. 2013; 9: 158–168.

Impact of Maternal Environment on Fetal Heart Rate

Ayona Wijemanne and Edwin Chandraharan

Introduction

The fetoplacental unit is a unique interface where oxygen is transferred to the fetus in exchange for carbon dioxide and water. Oxygen transfer is dependent upon adequate maternal oxygenation, uterine blood supply, placental transfer and integrity of the umbilical cord. Disruptions to any of these can result in fetal hypoxia and a subsequent change in fetal heart pattern on the CTG trace. Chemicals and inflammatory markers associated with maternal conditions may also cross the placenta and cause changes in fetal heart patterns. It is therefore important to consider the maternal environment when interpreting a cardiotocograph (CTH).

Key Facts

Maternal conditions or factors that may affect fetal heart patterns can be broadly categorized into the following groups:

Conditions Causing Maternal Metabolic Acidosis

- Diabetic ketoacidosis (DKA)
- Uraemic acidosis secondary to renal failure
- Starvation ketoacidosis
- Alcoholic ketoacidosis

Conditions Causing Chronic Maternal Hypoxia

- Maternal cardiovascular disease
  - Acquired/congenital cyanotic heart disease
  - Cardiac failure
  - Pulmonary hypertension
- Chronic pulmonary disease
  - Cystic fibrosis
- Severe maternal anaemia

Handbook of CTG Interpretation: From Patterns to Physiology, ed. Edwin Chandraharan. Published by Cambridge University Press. © Cambridge University Press 2017.

Conditions Reducing Placental Perfusion

This may lead to chronic hypoxia, as with:

- Preeclampsia
- Systemic lupus erythematosus

Placental perfusion may also be reduced temporarily with the following conditions:

- Maternal hypotension
- Maternal tachyarrhythmia

Maternal Autoantibodies

- Systemic lupus erythematosus
- Hyperthyroidism

Drugs

- Opiates (e.g. pethidine)
- Beta sympathomimetics (e.g. terbutaline)
- Cocaine

Maternal Temperature

Sepsis has already been discussed separately. However, there have been several case reports of maternal hypothermia (often resulting from sepsis) leading to prolonged decelerations on the CTG. This is corrected by rewarming the mother. Similarly, a fetus may react to maternal pyrexia by increasing its heart rate

Key Changes on the CTG Trace

Raised Baseline Fetal Heart Rate (FHR)

- Beta sympathomimetics (e.g. salbutamol or terbutaline)
- Fetal hyperthyroidism secondary to maternal anti-TSH receptor antibodies

Reduced Baseline FHR

- Congenital heart block secondary to maternal anti-Ro/La antibodies with SLE (Systemic Lupus Erythematosus); a baseline bradycardia may be noted.

Reduced Variability

- Chronic maternal hypoxia leading to chronic fetal hypoxic state
  - Severe maternal cardiac disease
- Conditions resulting in reduced placental perfusion, leading to chronic fetal hypoxic state
- Opiates
- Severe maternal metabolic acidosis

Chemoreceptor-Stimulated Decelerations
- Maternal metabolic acidosis

Prolonged Decelerations
- Maternal hypoglycaemia
- Maternal hypotension
- Maternal hypothermia

Key Pathophysiology behind the Features Observed on the CTG Trace

Raised Baseline FHR
- If present in significant titres, maternal anti-TSH receptor antibodies may cross the placenta and cause neonatal thyrotoxicosis. This manifests as a fetal tachycardia with a heart rate >160 bpm.
- Beta sympathomimetics cross the placenta and stimulate the fetal sympathetic nervous system, causing a fetal tachycardia.

Reduced Baseline FHR
- Maternal anti-Ro (SSA) and anti-La (SSB) antibodies cross the placenta and, if present in significant titres, cause inflammation of the fetal atrioventricular node and myocardium, resulting in congenital heart block.
- This occurs in 1–5 per cent of fetuses of mothers with SLE.
- The baseline FHR will typically be <100 bpm; NICE guidelines will not apply when interpreting such CTGs as this is a 'nonhypoxic' change in baseline FHR.

Reduced Variability
- Chronic maternal hypoxia and conditions resulting in reduced placental perfusion can cause intrauterine growth restriction and poor development of the fetal autonomic nervous system.
- Such fetuses will have reduced reserve and will not compensate for the hypoxic stress of labour as healthy fetuses; that is, reduced variability will appear on the CTG before the onset of decelerations and a rise in baseline.
- Opiates depress the fetal autonomic nervous system, resulting in reduced baseline variability.
- Maternal acidosis can reduce uterine blood flow and lead to decreased oxygenation of the fetoplacental unit. This change, along with the accumulation of maternal hydrogen ions in the fetus, may lead to fetal acidosis and subsequent reduced baseline variability. In these situations, variability may become reduced *before* the onset of decelerations.

Chemoreceptor-Simulated Decelerations

- Maternal metabolic acidosis leads to an increased maternal hydrogen ion concentration. These hydrogen ions cross the placenta and stimulate fetal chemoreceptors, causing shallow decelerations on the CTG trace.

Prolonged Decelerations

- Maternal hypotension is most commonly caused by aortocaval compression. Placental perfusion is reduced temporarily, causing a prolonged deceleration.

Management

Management of CTG abnormalities involves two principles:

- Correction of the precipitating cause
  - Relieving aortocaval compression by moving the mother into the left lateral position
  - Warming the mother in cases of hypothermia
- Considering the entire clinical picture
  - Threshold for delivery of growth-restricted fetuses will be much lower as they have less physiological reserve.

Key Tips for Optimizing the Outcome

- Anticipate problems beforehand
  - Fetal cardiac surveillance in mothers with anti-Ro/La antibodies
  - Regular growth scans in mothers with medical conditions causing chronic hypoxia
- A thorough assessment of the mother's medical condition on admission
  - Blood glucose and blood gas measurement in diabetic women with suspected DKA (Diabetic Ketoacidosis)
- A complete drug history including smoking and illicit drug use
- Timely correction of the precipitating factor(s)
- Anticipate a reactive fetal tachycardia for approximately 20 minutes after the administration of a tocolytic (e.g. terbutaline) for uterine hyperstimulation, and no intervention is necessary.

Common Pitfalls

- Proceeding directly to delivery by caesarean section in cases of prolonged decelerations secondary to maternal conditions rather than correcting the precipitating cause
- Misreading a baseline bradycardia as a prolonged deceleration
- Not considering the complete clinical picture

Consequences of Mismanagement

- Unnecessary operative deliveries
- Worsening of maternal medical condition (e.g. DKA) that, if left untreated, can lead to maternal death

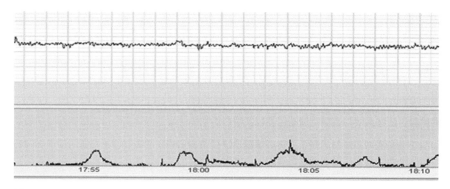

Figure 16.1

- Worsening fetal outcomes as attempting to perform an emergency caesarean section for a prolonged deceleration secondary to maternal hypotension may in fact worsen fetal outcome while increasing unnecessary operative interventions on the mother.

Exercise

1. A 31-year-old primigravida presents to the labour ward at 37 weeks of gestation with a history of regular contractions. She was diagnosed with type 1 diabetes at the age of 11 and uses insulin pump therapy. Her HBA1c at booking was 56 mmol/mol and control has been difficult during pregnancy. She appears dehydrated and urine dipstick shows >3 ketones. On admission she is found to be 3 cm dilated and CTG monitoring is commenced. The following trace is observed:
   a. How would you classify the CTG?
   b. What do you need to consider given her history and how might it impact upon the CTG?
   c. How will you manage her?

Further Reading

1. Hutter D, Kingdom J, Jaeggi E. Causes and mechanisms of intrauterine hypoxia and its impact on the fetal cardiovascular system: a review. *Int J Paeds.* 2010 (2010) 9.

2. Parker J, Conway D. Diabetic ketoacidosis in pregnancy. *Obstet Gynaec Clin NA.* 34 (2007) 533–543.

3. Aboud E, Neales K. The \effect of maternal hypothermia on the fetal heart rate. *Int J Obstet Gynecol.* 66 (1999) 163–164.

4. Balucan F, Morshed S, Davies T. Thyroid autoantibodies in pregnancy: their role, regulation and clinical relevance. *J Thyroid Res.* 2013 (2013) 15.

5. Jaeggi E, Laskin C, Hamilton R, Kingdom J. The importance of the level of maternal anti-Ro/SSA antibodies as a prognostic marker of the development of cardiac neonatal lupus erythematosus. *J Am Coll Cardiol.* 55 (2010) 2778–2784.

Chapter

17

Use of CTG with Induction and Augmentation of Labour

Ana Piñas Carrillo and Edwin Chandraharan

Key Facts

- The rates of both induction (IOL) and augmentation of labour are progressively increasing due to a better understanding of the course of obstetric and nonobstetric pathologies in pregnancy such as essential hypertension, preeclampsia, diabetes and obstetric cholestasis and improved and more widespread use of diagnostic techniques such as obstetric ultrasound to detect intrauterine growth restriction (IUGR) or fetal malformations that require an earlier delivery.

- The rate of IOL in the United Kingdom is around 20 per cent, similar to other developed countries, with 15 per cent of inductions requiring an instrumental delivery and 22 per cent an emergency caesarean section.

- Indications for IOL include maternal reasons such as preeclampsia, diabetes, obstetric cholestasis and other maternal diseases; fetal reasons include IUGR, multiple pregnancy and conditions inherent to the pregnancy such as prolonged rupture of membranes, meconium-stained liquor and postterm pregnancy.

- The most common method of IOL is the use of prostaglandin E2 in the form of pessary, tablet or gel. Other methods include the use of balloon catheter, oxytocin, prostaglandin E1 and antiprogesterons, the last two only licensed in cases of intrauterine death.

- Oxytocin and prostaglandins have no direct reported effects on the fetus, and their detrimental effects are mediated through excessive uterine activity and resultant compression of umbilical cord and/or reduction in oxygenation of placental venous sinuses.

- The most frequent complications occurring during the process of IOL are tachysystole, hypertonus or uterine hyperstimulation. Other complications include failed induction, rupture of membranes and occasionally umbilical cord prolapse, and uterine rupture especially in the presence of a previous uterine scar.

- Scientific evidence suggests that if the intercontraction interval is <2.3 minutes when oxytocin is used, there may be a rapid drop in oxygenated haemoglobin in the fetal brain.

Handbook of CTG Interpretation: From Patterns to Physiology, ed. Edwin Chandraharan. Published by Cambridge University Press. © Cambridge University Press 2017.

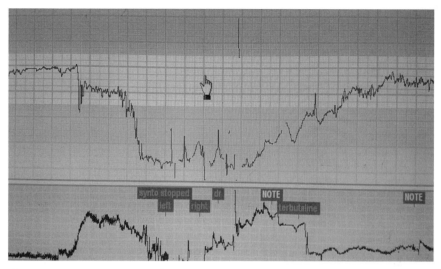

Figure 17.1 Note the occurrence of uterine hypertonus with no uterine relaxation.

Key Features on the CTG Trace

- 'Tachysystole' refers to the presence of five or more contractions in 10 minutes in the absence of changes in the FHR. Tachysystole requires careful observation until changes on the cardiograph are observed.
- 'Uterine hyperstimulation' refers to the presence of five or more contractions in 10 minutes (and/or increased tone and duration of uterine contractions), but, as opposed to tachysystole, it produces changes in the FHR. In early stages, typical variable decelerations appear; if excessive uterine activity (frequency, duration or strength) continues, the CTG may show atypical and late decelerations (secondary to reduction in utero-placental oxygenation), rise in baseline heart rate and loss of variability ('gradually evolving hypoxia').
- 'Hypertonia' or 'uterine hypertonus' refers to a sustained uterine contraction lasting >60 seconds and has the potential to cause a prolonged deceleration (Figure 17.1). In cases of previous caesarean section, this can reflect a uterine rupture (see Chapter 15.)

Key Pathophysiology behind Patterns Seen on the CTG Trace

- An evolving uterine hyperstimulation usually produces features suggestive of a 'gradually evolving hypoxia' on the CTG trace (decelerations followed by an absence of accelerations, rise in baseline FHR initially followed by a loss of baseline variability and a 'stepladder' pattern to death due to the onset of decompensation).
- A rapidly evolving or sustained uterine contraction may cause an acute umbilical cord compression leading to a prolonged deceleration caused by an acute interruption of fetal oxygenation. This prolonged deceleration is usually characterized by the presence of good variability within the first 3 minutes of deceleration (in the absence of three major accidents: abruption, uterine rupture and cord prolapse). However, if it is not rapidly treated, variability may subsequently disappear suggestive of hypoxia to the centres in the brain that control FHR.

Recommended Management

- In the presence of uterine hyperstimulation, prostaglandins should be removed or oxytocin should be stopped immediately if labour is being augmented. If CTG changes persist with no signs of normalization, tocolytics (terbutaline 250 mcg subcutaneously) should be administered to relax uterine myometrium and to relieve umbilical cord compression and replenish oxygenation of placental venous sinuses so as to ensure adequate fetal oxygenation. As soon as the uterine activity is reduced, the CTG trace should show signs of recovery, with decelerations becoming narrower and shallower and a progressive reduction of fetal heart baseline to the initial rate due to a reduction in catecholamine surge and improvement of baseline variability (if it was reduced in response to hyperstimulation).
- If there is a tachysystole, there is no need to intervene, but if there are any other risk factors such as a previous uterine scar, IUGR or meconium-stained liquor among others, the same management as with uterine hyperstimulation should be considered to avoid further complications (i.e. uterine rupture, meconium aspiration syndrome or rapid fetal compromise in IUGR due to a reduced physiological reserve).
- If there is a prolonged deceleration secondary to a sustained contraction, removal of prostaglandins or stoppage of oxytocin infusion are immediate interventions. If there are no attempts at recovery of FHR to its original baseline, administration of tocolytics should be considered. In the absence of three major accidents (abruption, cord prolapse and uterine rupture), the '3, 6, 9, 12, 15' rule can be applied. In this clinical scenario, 90 per cent of prolonged decelerations recover to normal baseline in 6 minutes and up to 95 per cent in 9 minutes, once the offending agent (prostaglandin or oxytocin) is removed and tocolytics were administered (if indicated).

Key Tips to Optimize Outcome

- Individualize every case and appropriately select the method and suitability of IOL/augmentation. A severely compromised IUGR fetus with redistribution is unlikely to have sufficient physiological reserves to cope with the process of IOL.
- During augmentation of labour, in the presence of early signs of gradually evolving hypoxia (variable decelerations, absence of accelerations), anticipate further changes and review the need to continue increasing oxytocin if regular contractions have been achieved. One may need to re-examine a woman in 2 hours instead of 4 hours to assess the progress of labour, because if there is evidence of progress, further increments of oxytocin dosage are not necessary.
- Remember that as labour progresses, the number of oxytocin receptors increases in the fundus, making the myometrium more sensitive to circulating oxytocin, and therefore, less oxytocin may be needed as labour advances.
- Current scientific evidence suggests that the use of oxytocin to augment spontaneous labour reduces the mean duration of labour by approximately 2 hours without influencing the mode of birth. Therefore, in the light of this evidence, caution should be exercised in the use of oxytocin in high-risk labour (previous caesarean section, IUGR, meconium, clinical chorioamnionitis) as the benefit of 2-hour reduction in the duration of labour may not outweigh the risks of uterine rupture, fetal

hypoxic-ischaemic injury, synergistic hypoxic neurological damage in chorioamnionitis or meconium aspiration syndrome.

- If oxytocin is restarted, the lowest possible dose to ensure optimum uterine contractions should be used. For practical purposes, half the dose that resulted in uterine hyperstimulation should be tried, if appropriate.
- During second stage of labour, oxytocin should be used with great caution as uterine myometrium is maximally sensitive to oxytocin during this time and injudicious use of oxytocin may result in rapidly evolving hypoxia and fetal neurological injury.

Pitfalls

- Failure to incorporate the clinical picture into the management. The presence of meconium-stained liquor, chorioamnionitis or IUGR should be taken into account when considering augmentation of labour. In the presence of any of these risk factors, increasing the hypoxic stress can have dramatic consequences on the fetus.
- Interrupting the process of IOL in the presence of a tachysystole. In the absence of fetal compromise, there is no need to remove prostaglandins or administer tocolytics.
- Injudicious use of oxytocin especially only concentrating on the frequency of uterine contractions without considering uterine activity (frequency, duration and strength).
- Failure to ensure adequate intercontraction interval to facilitate optimal oxygenation of placental venous sinuses when oxytocin is used to induce or augment labour.

Consequences of Mismanagement

- Meconium aspiration syndrome with increased perinatal morbidity and mortality
- Intrapartum stillbirth
- Neonatal death
- Hypoxic-ischaemic encephalopathy
- Uterine rupture
- Unnecessary operative interventions

Exercise

1. A 30-year-old, G2 P1, previous caesarean section is being induced for postdates (41 + 4 weeks of gestation). She had prostaglandin pessary inserted for 24 hours, following which she had an artificial rupture of membranes (ARMs) that showed meconium grade 1. Two hours later, she was started on oxytocin infusion. Oxytocin has been augmented every 30 minutes as per protocol. CTG trace before the ARM was normal with a baseline FHR of 130 bpm, variability of 10–15 bpm, presence of accelerations with no decelerations and she had two contractions in 10 minutes.
   CTG after 8 hours of oxytocin augmentation shows the following features:
   a. What is your diagnosis?
   b. What is your management?
   c. What other complications do you expect?

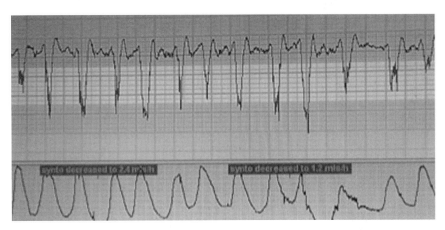

Figure 17.2

Further Reading

1. McCarthy FP, Kenny LC. Induction of labour. *Obstet, Gynaecol, Reprod Med.* 2013; 24(1): 9–15.

2. National Institute for Health and Clinical Excellence. *Induction of labour. Clinical guideline 70.* Available at www.nice.org.uk/CG070; July 2008.

3. *WHO recommendations for augmentation of labour.* 2014

4. McDonnell S, Chandraharan E. The pathophysiology of CTGs and types of intrapartum hypoxia. *Curr Women's Health Rev.* 2013; 9: 158–168.

5. Chandraharan E, Arulkumaran S. Acute tocolysis. *Curr Opin Obstet Gynecol.* 2005; 17: 151–156.

Recognition of Chronic Hypoxia and the Preterminal Cardiotocograph

Austin Ugwumadu

The Fetal Neurologic State

- A normal developing fetus exhibits a range of often coordinated and rhythmical behavioural states including gross movements, eye movements and fetal heart rate (FHR). An underlying assumption in studying these variables is that they may reflect fetal brain development and that factors that impair brain development or function may lead to abnormalities in the clustering of these variables, their occurrence and/ or their qualitative appearance. One such factor is chronic hypoxia, and its effect on the general characteristics of FHR, in particular FHR variability, forms the basis of recognition of fetuses with an antecedent injury.

- Although there are marked interfetal variations in the normal neurologic state, the term and near-term fetus may spend up to 25 per cent of its time in quiet (non–rapid eye movement [REM] sleep) during which FHR, fetal heart variability and movements are reduced.[1] Near term, quiet sleep lasts for approximately 20 minutes and active sleep approximately 40 minutes.[2] The mechanisms that control these cycles of rest and activity in the fetus are yet to be fully elucidated.

Physiology of FHR Regulation and Variability

- Baseline FHR is the summation of moment-by-moment autonomic modulation from the medullary cardiorespiratory centre in response to an array of inputs from (a) chemoreceptors, (b) baroreceptors, (c) hormonal regulation, (d) central nervous system activities such as sleep and arousal states and (e) blood volume control. The parasympathetic innervation of the heart originates from the medulla oblongata through the vagus nerve to supply the sinoatrial (SA) and atrioventricular (AV) nodal pacemaker tissues where on stimulation it exerts two main effects, namely, reduction in the rate of firing of the SA nodal tissue resulting in a fall in FHR, and an oscillatory effect which alters the R-wave intervals resulting in FHR variability.

- There is no regulatory vagal innervation to the myocardium. Vagotomy or administration of atropine will block the release of acetylcholine from the vagus nerve endings at the SA node with a resultant increase in FHR. Sympathetic nervous system fibres, on the other hand, are widely distributed throughout the myocardium of the term fetus. Stimulation releases noradrenaline at the nerve endings resulting in an increase in FHR, contractility and cardiac output. The administration of

Handbook of CTG Interpretation: From Patterns to Physiology, ed. Edwin Chandraharan. Published by Cambridge University Press. © Cambridge University Press 2017.

sympathoplegics or lesions of sympathetic pathway results in a fall in baseline FHR and blunt FHR accelerations.

- FHR variability represents slight differences in time intervals between each heartbeat and the next (aka short-term variability) as counted and recorded by the heart rate monitor. If these intervals were identical, the FHR trace would be straight, smooth and regular. Although this beat-to-beat variability is frequently and loosely attributed to the interactions between sympathetic and parasympathetic reflexes, the facts are much more complex than that.

- The source of FHR variability includes input from cerebral cortex, midbrain, vagus nerve and specialized cardiac pacemaker tissues. That final FHR variability is due to beat-to-beat adjustments from baroreceptor influence, or from rapidly oscillating vagal impulses, which vary irregularly in frequency and amplitude and involve short- and long-term changes.[3,4] The magnitude of FHR variability may be affected by fetal breathing, fetal movements and fetal sleep state.

- In practice, FHR variability is observed as irregular fluctuations in amplitude and frequency of baseline FHR on a CTG paper and quantified as the amplitude of peak-to-trough in beats per minute. To exhibit a normal FHR variability, the fetus requires an intact cerebral cortex, midbrain, vagus nerve and cardiac conductive tissues.

- FHR variability has emerged as a critical determinant of adequate perfusion, oxygenation and function of the central nervous system and the FHR characteristic most consistently associated with new-born acidosis and morbidity. Even in the presence of decelerations or bradycardia, a fetus that displays a normal variability has a very low risk of acidaemia, immediate death or asphyxial brain injury,[5-7] while absent or reduced variability was associated with significant new-born acidaemia in both term[7,8] and preterm infants.[9] In a recent systematic review, minimal or undetectable FHR variability was the most consistent predictor of new-born acidaemia.[5] In contrast, increased FHR variation was observed in association with severe acidosis and hypotension in a hypoxia-ischaemia model using term-equivalent fetal sheep.[10] Furthermore, absent FHR variability may be idiopathic, but usually the other features of FHR are normal, including cycling activity and absence of FHR decelerations.

Fetal Response to Hypoxia-Ischaemia

- Under normal conditions, a large number of control mechanisms are activated in response to acute hypoxia including chemoreceptor, baroreceptor, sympathetic and parasympathetic influences. Therefore, fetal response to hypoxia-ischaemia is complex. For the purposes of this chapter, it suffices to state the following well-established observations: fetal response to maternal hypoxia, reduced uterine blood flow, or to an umbilical cord occlusion is a prompt FHR deceleration. This deceleration has a drop of approximately 30 bpm from the original baseline. This deceleration (or bradycardia) depending on the duration of insult is variably associated with hypertension and, therefore, can occur with baroreceptor as well as chemoreceptor activation.

- In the absence of progressive acidaemia, the fetal sheep may restore its FHR and variability to normal after approximately 12–16 hours of exposure to acute hypoxia. In addition to FHR deceleration outlined above, initial response to hypoxia includes a rise in fetal blood pressure, a rapid and up to 60 per cent reduction in oxygen consumption, which can be sustained for up to 45 minutes depending on the degree of hypoxia and rapidly reversible if the insult is removed and oxygenation restored. A further response is adrenergic activation. The resultant β-adrenergic activity leads to increased inotropic effect to maintain or increase cardiac output and umbilical blood flow, while the α-adrenergic activity is important in determining regional blood flow in the hypoxic fetus by selective vasoconstriction. The 60 per cent reduction in oxygen consumption, FHR deceleration/bradycardia, anaerobic glycolysis and selective vasoconstriction enable the fetus to survive a relatively long period of limited oxygen supply currently estimated to be approximately 30–60 minutes without damage to vital organs. If hypoxia persists, metabolic acidosis would develop due to lactic acid accumulation in those organs where there has been vasoconstriction and inadequate oxygen supply for metabolic needs, and in severe or sustained cases, the above responses fail and are followed by a decline in cardiac output, blood pressure and blood flow to the brain.

FHR Characteristics of a Chronically Hypoxic Fetus

- The admission CTG may be controversial; however, a prompt recognition of the fetus with a preexisting brain injury in early labour is one of the strongest arguments in its favour. Such a key finding permits the obstetrician and/or the midwife to assign or reassign the patient to her appropriate risk category. A normal CTG is the hallmark of fetal well-being,[11] suggests normoxia,[12] normal acid–base status,[13,14] absence of asphyxia[13,14] and, in the absence of unpredictable obstetric catastrophe, a low probability of intrapartum fetal asphyxia.[15]

- A normal CTG also suggests that the fetal neurological and cardiovascular systems are intact and able to react and defend the fetus against intrapartum insults. In contrast, the fetus with an abnormal CTG in early labour may already be injured and is likely to exhibit maladaptive or no compensatory responses if exposed to asphyxiating insults during labour. Such a fetus is at risk of adverse outcome,[15] including intrapartum death and long-term neurological deficits.[16–18]

- Fetuses with antecedent brain injury from hypoxic-ischaemic insults do not exhibit a uniform set of FHR patterns during labour. However, they do display distinct FHR patterns, which allow the clinician to profile their risk and management on the basis of initial FHR on admission and subsequent changes in baseline FHR. The characteristic, but by no means exclusive, FHR pattern of antenatally injured fetus is nonreactive CTG with a fixed and invariable baseline from admission to delivery, associated with reduced or average FHR variability[16,17,19] (Figure 18.1). This pattern does not suggest an ongoing asphyxial insult but represents a post–brain injury compensatory response by the fetus, a sort of static intrauterine encephalopathy.

- In a study of 300 brain-damaged babies who were monitored on admission in labour, a persistently nonreactive FHR pattern was found in 45 per cent.[17] Phelan and Kim categorized these nonreactive admission CTGs into three groups on the basis of baseline FHR and FHR variability in order to correlate the FHR patterns to the duration of time from injury.[20] They concluded that fetuses admitted with FHR tachycardia >160 bpm and reduced or absent variability were likely to be closer to the time of insult compared to their peers with normal baseline FHR and reduced or even average FHR variability who are likely to be further remote from the time of brain injury.

(a)

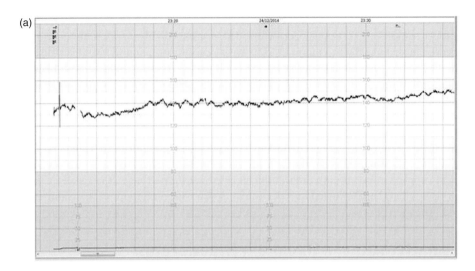

(b)

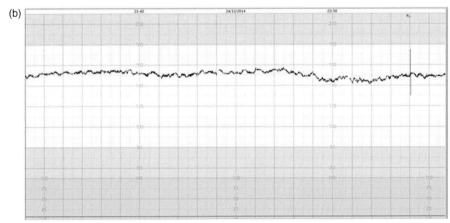

(c)

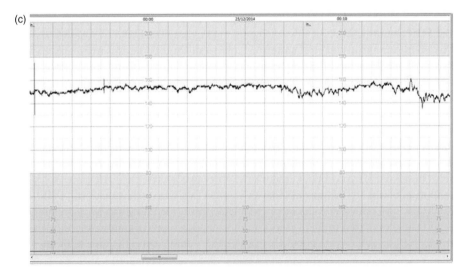

(d)

(e)

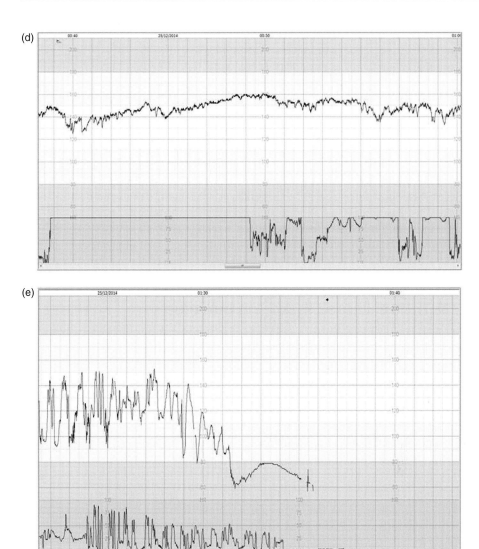

Figure 18.1 Parous woman, with uneventful antenatal course, admitted with spontaneous early labour at 38 + 5 weeks of gestation. She was started on CTG because FHR decelerations were heard on intermittent auscultation. The CTG showed typical nonreactive FHR pattern with reduced variability of antenatal fetal injury. She delivered spontaneously many hours later with FHR collapse in the second stage of labour. Apgar score 1 and 1 at 1 and 5 minutes, arterial pH 6.9, venous pH 7.0, HIE grade 3. This outcome is inconsistent with the gases. MRI showed symmetrical signal abnormality in the thalami and to a lesser extent in basal ganglia and hippocampi. (A) CTG trace on admission shows absence of baseline variability. (B) Continuation of the CTG trace shows absence of cycling. (C) CTG continues to show a higher-than-expected baseline FHR for a posttermfetus. (D) CTG trace shows the appearance of 'shallow decelerations' with advancing labour. (E) CTG trace shows the onset of a terminal bradycardia which is the end stage of chronic hypoxia leading to an acute on chronic insult.

- Tachycardia associated with a 'gradually evolving hypoxia' may still be in evolution when a woman presents in labour, and this pattern may mimic the chronically hypoxic fetus. The clinician may be confused because he or she did not observe the previously normal FHR pattern. However, this pattern is, by definition, almost always accompanied by repetitive complex variable decelerations. Once tachycardia begins in response to repetitive decelerations, the natural history of this pattern may lead to one of a number of outcomes, namely, FHR tachycardia persists or continues to rise until delivery, or a prolonged and persistent FHR deceleration or bradycardia until delivery, or slow but progressive decline of FHR from tachycardia as the fetus approaches death. In this specific subset of fetuses, the value of FHR variability as a reliable indicator of fetal well-being has been challenged.[21] A proportion of brain-damaged children exhibited average FHR variability at the time of their delivery and manifested cerebral oedema in the neonatal period suggesting that brain injury in this context may precede loss of FHR variability.

- One relevant question is how FHR variability was defined in that study. In practice, increased FHR variation associated with severe acidosis may be abrupt, erratic, high amplitude, and lack the natural wavelike characteristic of normal FHR variability and are oftentimes still classified as increased FHR variability or saltatory patterns. This is incorrect as it implies exaggerated but normal wavelike variability.

Other Markers of Chronic Hypoxia in the Fetus

- Other markers of chronic hypoxia and fetal compromise may be observed in these cases, including reduced fetal movement prior to admission, oligohydramnios, presence of old meconium staining of amniotic fluid, meconium aspiration syndrome and subsequent pulmonary hypertension. Meconium is known to induce vasoconstriction of fetoplacental and chorionic vessels and in high concentrations may cause ulcerations of these vessels.[22,23] In addition, meconium degrades the bacteriostatic activity of the amniotic fluid, thereby increasing the risk of ascending infection and chorioamnionitis.[24,25]

- Therefore, it is conceivable that at least a proportion of the fetuses with meconium contamination of the amniotic fluid are possibly in a state of systemic vasoconstriction and may be vulnerable to decompensation and brain injury during labour. Furthermore, fetuses with a fixed nonreactive FHR pattern have raised nucleated red blood cells (NRBCs),[26,27] prolonged NRBC clearance times,[26] low platelet counts,[28] delayed onset of seizures from birth,[29] multiorgan system dysfunction[30] and cortical brain injuries.[17]

The Preterminal CTG

- The definition of preterminal CTG in classic textbooks and teaching modules, involving FHR tachycardia, reduced or absent variability and shallow FHR decelerations, may be misleading in clinical practice. First, the reason such end-stage FHR patterns are classified as 'preterminal' is because the fetus is at risk of death if it is not delivered expeditiously. However, there are several other FHR patterns, which, if left to run their natural courses, would also result in fetal demise without necessarily operating via the widely recognized and reported preterminal CTG pattern.

- These other patterns include prolonged and persistent FHR deceleration or bradycardia, particularly if associated with a loss of FHR variability, tachycardia associated with FHR deceleration and loss of variability, and severe subacute hypoxia pattern in which there are high amplitude and long-standing FHR decelerations and short interdeceleration intervals. Clinicians should rethink their definition and approach to FHR patterns, which carry the risk of intrapartum fetal death.

Conclusions

- A prompt recognition of the FHR pattern of chronically hypoxic fetus and preterminal CTG is essential to initiating appropriate and timely intervention to achieve a good outcome. Typically, the fetus with antecedent brain injury exhibits a nonreactive CTG with a fixed and nonvariable baseline associated with reduced or average variability, which should not be confused with ongoing asphyxial insult but represents a postinjury static encephalopathy.

- Fetuses admitted with FHR tachycardia >160 bpm and reduced or absent variability are likely to have suffered a recent injury, in contrast to their peers with normal baseline FHR and reduced or average FHR variability who are likely to be remote from the time of brain injury.

References

1. Manning FA. Assessment of fetal condition and risk: analysis of single and combined biophysical variable monitoring. *Semin Perinatol*. 1985;9:168–83.

2. Van Woerdeen EE, VanGeijn HP. Heart rate patterns and FMs. In J. Nijhuis (ed.) *Fetal Behaviour*. New York, NY: Oxford University Press; 1992:41.

3. Parer JT. Fetal heart rate. In R.K. Creasy, R. Resnik, JD Iams (eds.) *Maternal Fetal Medicine: Principles and Practice* (5th ed). Philadelphia: Saunders; 2004.

4. Parer JTP, King TL. Whither fetal heart rate monitoring? *Obstet Gynecol Fertil*. 1999;22:149.

5. Parer JT, King T, Flanders S, Fox M, Kilpatrick SJ. Fetal acidaemia and electronic fetal heart rate patterns: is there evidence of an association? *J Matern Fetal Neonatal Med*. 2006;19:289–94.

6. Young BK, Katz M, Klein SA, Silverman F. Fetal blood and tissue pH with moderate bradycardia. *Am J Obstet Gynecol*. 1979;135:45–7.

7. Williams KP, Galerneau F. Fetal heart rate parameters predictive of neonatal outcome in the presence of a prolonged deceleration. *Obstet Gynecol*. 2002;100:951–4.

8. Williams KP, Galerneau F. Intrapartum fetal heart rate patterns in the prediction of neonatal acidemia. *Am J Obstet Gynecol*. 2003;188:820–3.

9. Matsuda Y, Maeda T, Kouno S. The critical period of non-reassuring fetal heart rate patterns in preterm gestation. *Eur J Obstet Gynecol Reprod Biol*. 2003;106:36–9.

10. Westgate JA, Bennet L, Gunn AJ. Fetal heart rate variability changes during brief repeated umbilical cord occlusion in near term fetal sheep. *Br J Obstet Gynaecol*. 1999;106:664–71.

11. Phelan JP. Labour admission test. *Clin Perinatol*. 1994;21:879–85.

12. Carbonne B, Langer B, Goffinet F, Audibert F, Tardif D, Le Goueff F. et al. Multicenter study on the clinical value of fetal pulse oximetry. II. Compared predictive values of pulse oximetry and fetal blood analysis. The French Study Group on Fetal Pulse Oximetry. *Am J Obstet Gynecol*. 1997;177:593–8.

13. Clark SL, Gimovsky ML, Miller FC. The scalp stimulation test: a clinical alternative to fetal scalp blood sampling. *Am J Obstet Gynecol*. 1984;148:274–7.

14. Shaw K, Clark SL. Reliability of intrapartum fetal heart rate monitoring in the postterm fetus with meconium passage. *Obstet Gynecol*. 1988;72:886–9.

15. Ingemarsson I, Arulkumaran S, Ingemarsson E, Tambyraja RL, Ratnam SS. Admission test: a screening test for

fetal distress in labor. *Obstet Gynecol.* 1986;68:800–6.

16. Phelan JP, Ahn MO. Perinatal observations in forty-eight neurologically impaired term infants. *Am J Obstet Gynecol.* 1994;171:424–31.

17. Phelan JP, Ahn MO. Fetal heart rate observations in 300 term brain-damaged infants. *J Matern Fetal Inv.* 1998;8:1–5.

18. Devoe LD, McKenzie J, Searle NS, Sherline DM. Clinical sequelae of the extended nonstress test. *Am J Obstet Gynecol.* 1985;151:1074–8.

19. Leveno KJ, Williams ML, DePalma RT, Whalley PJ. Perinatal outcome in the absence of antepartum fetal heart rate acceleration. *Obstet Gynecol.* 1983;61:347–55.

20. Phelan JP, Kim JO. Fetal heart rate observations in the brain-damaged infant. *Semin Perinatol.* 2000;24:221–9.

21. Takahashi Y, Ukita M, Nakada E. Intrapartum FHR monitoring and neonatal CT brain scan. *Nihon Sanka Fujinka Gakkai Zasshi.* 1982;34:2133–42.

22. Altshuler G, Arizawa M, Molnar-Nadasdy G. Meconium-induced umbilical cord vascular necrosis and ulceration: a potential link between the placenta and poor pregnancy outcome. *Obstet Gynecol.* 1992;79:760–6.

23. Pickens J, Toubas PL, Hyde S, Altshuler G. In vitro model of human umbilical venous perfusion to study the effects of meconium staining of the umbilical cord. *Biol Neonate.* 1995;67:100–8.

24. Perlman JM, Risser R, Broyles RS. Bilateral cystic periventricular leukomalacia in the premature infant: associated risk factors. *Pediatrics.* 1996;97:822–7.

25. Yoon BH, Romero R, Kim CJ, Jun JK, Gomez R, Choi JH, Syn HC. Amniotic fluid interleukin-6: a sensitive test for antenatal diagnosis of acute inflammatory lesions of preterm placenta and prediction of perinatal morbidity. *Am J Obstet Gynecol.* 1995;172:960–70.

26. Phelan JP, Ahn MO, Korst LM, Martin GI. Nucleated red blood cells: a marker for fetal asphyxia? *Am J Obstet Gynecol.* 1995;173:1380–4.

27. Buonocore G, Perrone S, Gioia D, Gatti MG, Massafra C, Agosta R. et al. Nucleated red blood cell count at birth as an index of perinatal brain damage. *Am J Obstet Gynecol.* 1999;181:1500–5.

28. Korst LM, Phelan JP, Wang YM, Ahn MO. Neonatal platelet counts in fetal brain injury. *Am J Perinatol.* 1999;16:79–83.

29. Ahn MO, Korst LM, Phelan JP, Martin GI. Does the onset of neonatal seizures correlate with the timing of fetal neurologic injury? *Clin Pediatr* (Phila). 1998;37:673–6.

30. Korst LM, Phelan JP, Wang YM, Martin GI, Ahn MO. Acute fetal asphyxia and permanent brain injury: a retrospective analysis of current indicators. *J Matern Fetal Med.* 1999;8:101–6.

Chapter

19

Unusual Fetal Heart Rate Patterns
Sinusoidal and Saltatory Patterns

Madhusree Ghosh and Edwin Chandraharan

Key Facts

- A sinusoidal (typical) fetal heart rate (FHR) pattern may be due to physiological causes like fetal thumb sucking or administration of narcotic analgesics like alphaprodine[2,3] and butorphanol.[4,5]
- The most common pathological cause of sinusoidal FHR is fetal anaemia due to rhesus isoimmunization (typical sinusoidal pattern) with fetal hypoxia and acidosis and sudden loss of fetal blood volume due to acute fetomaternal haemorrhage (atypical sinusoidal pattern).
- Saltatory FHR patterns[6] can be due to uterine hyperstimulation, ephedrine administration and repeated intensive hypoxic stress such as active maternal pushing in active second stage of labour.

Key Features on the CTG Trace

Features of sinusoidal heart rate are:

- Stable baseline FHR of 120 to 160 beats per minute with regular sine-wave oscillations
- Amplitude of 5 to 15 beats per minute
- Frequency of 2 to 5 cycles per minute
- Reduced or absent baseline variability
- Absence of accelerations

The features of saltatory pattern are (see Figure 19.2):

- Fetal heart rate baseline amplitude changes greater than 25 beats per minute
- Oscillatory frequency of greater than 6 per minute
- Minimum duration of 1 minute

Sinusoidal FHR can be further classified as[7]:

- Smooth or typical – rounded, symmetric in shape
- Jagged or atypical – jagged, saw-toothed form, also termed as 'Poole shark teeth pattern' (Figure 19.1)
- Pseudo-sinusoidal – undulatory waveforms or regular FHR baseline oscillations of constant amplitude, alternating with episodes of normal baseline variability and reactivity

Handbook of CTG Interpretation: From Patterns to Physiology, ed. Edwin Chandraharan. Published by Cambridge University Press. © Cambridge University Press 2017.

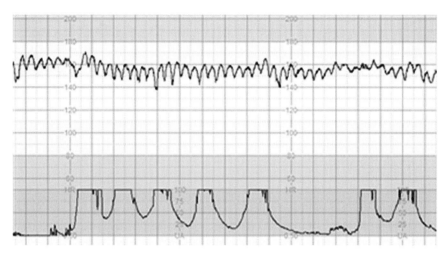

Figure 19.1 Atypical sinusoidal pattern: 'Poole shark teeth pattern'.

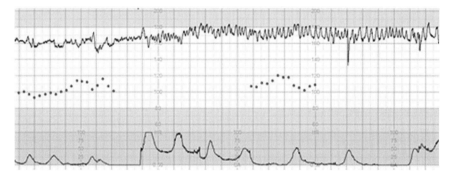

Figure 19.2 Pseudo-sinusoidal pattern. Note the presence of normal variability prior to sinusoidal pattern.

Key Pathophysiology of Sinusoidal and Saltatory FHR Patterns

- Exact pathophysiology not well understood due to its rare occurrence.
- Sinusoidal FHR is either due to central nervous system involvement or an umbilical cord–related aetiology such as acute and repeated umbilical cord compression leading to alternative episodes of fetal hypovolemia and hypertension.
- Derangement or loss of central nervous system control over the FHR is believed to be the common pathway of sinusoidal FHR patterns. This may explain the occurrence of this pattern after administration of certain drugs that act on the central nervous system and fetal hypoxia and acidosis.
- Sinusoidal FHR pattern may occur due to a massive fetomaternal transfusion and maternal anaemia. Severe anaemia may lead to local relative hypoxia of specialized tissues such as the central nervous system cardiac centre leading to sinusoidal pattern.
- Sinusoidal FHR is also seen in the presence of chorioamnionitis. The fetuses may not be hypoxic but show a sinusoidal FHR pattern due to maternal pyrexia. This is because elevated maternal temperature may adversely affect fetal brain function, thereby inactivating central nervous system control over FHR.

- Atypical sinusoidal pattern is believed to occur secondary to acute fetal hypotension and resultant acute hypoxia to the central nervous system that causes instability of the autonomic nervous system.
- Pseudo-sinusoidal FHR is not typically associated with fetal compromise.
- Saltatory FHR is probably a result of instability between sympathetic and parasympathetic nervous systems resulting in rapidly evolving hypoxia to the central nervous system.

Recommended Management

- Exclude predisposing causes for sinusoidal and saltatory patterns.
- Sinusoidal traces secondary to administration of drugs can be managed expectantly.
- Due to a lack of correlation between sinusoidal traces and documented fetal hypoxia, one needs to consider the underlying clinical picture, for example, reduced fetal movement, presence of meconium, intrapartum bleeding prior to embarking on operative delivery.
- An ultrasound scan may be performed to confirm fetal thumb sucking.
- In cases of typical or atypical sinusoidal traces for >10 minutes in the presence of risk factors (Rhesus-negative status, sudden fetomaternal bleeding), urgent delivery is indicated by the quickest and safest mode of birth.
- In cases of saltatory patterns, oxytocin infusion should be reduced or stopped and the woman should be advised to stop pushing in the second stage of labour to improve utero-placental circulation and re-establish oxygenation of the brain. If improvement in the features of CTG trace are observed, labour may be allowed to continue. If saltatory pattern persists despite conservative measures and immediate delivery is not imminent, tocolysis should be continued. Delivery should be accomplished if there is no improvement despite intrauterine resuscitation.
- The neonatal team should be notified as the neonate may be hypoxic or hypotensive at birth requiring advanced neonatal resuscitation and blood transfusion.

Key Tips to Optimize Outcome

- Unusual FHR patterns may be physiological; however, pathological causes need to be excluded.
- Exclude predisposing factors such as chronic fetal anaemia, chorioamnionitis and administration of drugs to the mother.
- Prompt recognition of sinusoidal pattern where there is an ongoing fetomaternal haemorrhage is essential.
- Clear communication with multidisciplinary team is mandatory.
- Escalate and seek immediate senior obstetric help when unsure about unusual patterns.
- Continuous training of obstetric doctors and midwives on unusual FHR patterns, their significance and management is recommended.

Pitfalls

- Failure to differentiate between physiological and persisting sinusoidal patterns due to ongoing fetomaternal haemorrhage.

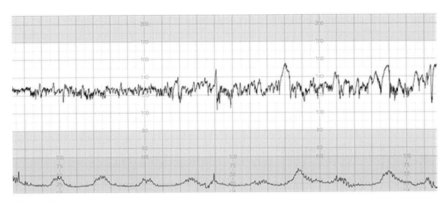

Figure 19.3

- Failure to recognize concealed placental abruption and ongoing atypical sinusoidal pattern.
- Failure to inform the neonatal team regarding the possibility of severe fetal anaemia and/or hypotension, which may require an urgent neonatal blood transfusion after birth.

Consequences of Mismanagement

- Intrapartum fetal death and early neonatal death.
- Severe hypoxic-ischaemic encephalopathy (HIE).
- Unnecessary operative intervention due to lack of recognition and treatment of a sinusoidal pattern secondary to a physiological cause.
- Maternal hypotension and disseminated intravascular coagulopathy (DIC) due to a failure of recognition of an atypical sinusoidal pattern secondary to a concealed abruption.

Exercise

1. A 35-year-old primigravida presents at 38 weeks of gestation with abdominal pain for 3 hours and reduced fetal movements with no vaginal bleeding. On examination, uterine contractions were palpated and the cervix was fully effaced, 2 cm dilated.
   a. What is your differential diagnosis?
   b. Is a CTG indicated?
   c. She was re-examined in 4 hours and established to be in labour. She was later commenced on oxytocin for confirmed delay in the first stage of labour. Vaginal examination after 4 hours of oxytocin demonstrated that she was 8 cm dilated. Describe the CTG at this stage (Figure 19.3). Do you have any concerns?
   d. She opted for an epidural anesthesia and is now fully dilated and has had a 2-hour passive descent. A repeat vaginal examination suggests that she is fully dilated with the fetal head in occipito-anterior position, at station +1. A decision has been made to start active pushing. She has been actively pushing for 20 minutes and CTG is given below (Figure 19.4). How would you describe the CTG?
   e. What is your management plan based on the features observed on the CTG (Figure 19.4)?

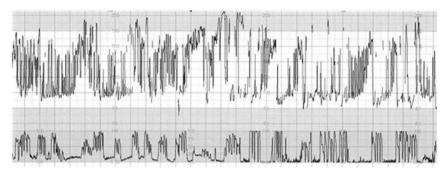

Figure 19.4

References

1. *The Use of Electronic Fetal Monitoring.* London: National Institute for Clinical Excellence; 2001.

2. Gray JH, Cudmore DW, Luther ER, Martin TR, Gardner AJ. Sinusoidal fetal heart rate pattern associated with alphaprodine administration. *Obstet Gynecol* 1978;52:678–81.

3. Veren D, Boehm FH, Killam AP. The clinical significance of sinusoidal fetal heart rate pattern associated with alphaprodine administration. *J Reprod Med* 1982;27:411–4.

4. Angel JL, Knuppel RA, Lake M. Sinusoidal fetal heart rate pattern associated with intravenous butorphanol administration: a case report. *Am J Obstet Gynecol* 1984;149:465–7.

5. Hatjis CG, Meis PJ. Sinusoidal fetal heart rate pattern associated with butorphanol administration. *Obstet Gynecol* 1986;67:377–80.

6. Yanamandra N, Chandraharan E. Saltatory and sinusoidal fetal heart rate patterns and significance of FHR 'overshoots'. *Curr Women's Health Rev.* 2013;9:175–82.

7. Graca LM, Cardoso CG, Calhaz-jorge C. An approach to interpretation and classification of sinusoidal fetal heart rate patterns. *Eur J Obstet Gynecol Reprod Biol* 1988;27:203–12.

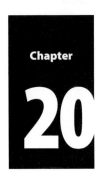

Chapter

20

Intrauterine Resuscitation

Abigail Spring and Edwin Chandraharan

Key Facts

- Intrauterine resuscitation is easy to perform and can result in a significant improvement in the in-utero fetal condition.
- The reversal of fetal hypoxia and acidosis may allow labour to continue safely or optimize the fetal condition/well-being until urgent delivery is accomplished. If not corrected, it may result in fetal decompensation leading to hypoxic injury.
- Oxygen delivery to the fetus is dependent on:
  - Uterine oxygen delivery: maternal haemoglobin, oxygen saturation and perfusion pressure, maternal position.
  - Utero-placental circulation: uterine activity (frequency, duration and strength of contractions), size of 'placental pools'.
  - Transfer of oxygen to the fetus: cord compression, cord prolapse.
  - Fetal circulation: high fetal haemoglobin concentration, fetal cardiac output highly dependent on fetal heart rate (FHR).

Key Features on the CTG Trace

- 'Fetal distress' is a nonspecific term used to describe concerns on the CTG trace, and therefore, clinicians should instead use the term 'suspected fetal compromise'.
- Decelerations – these may be early, variable, late or prolonged (>3 minutes).
- Fetal bradycardia (<110 bpm persisting for >10 minutes).
- Uterine hyperstimulation (increased frequency, strength or duration of contractions associated with CTG changes).
- Loss of baseline variability with preceding decelerations and rise in baseline FHR.

Key Pathophysiology behind Patterns Seen on the CTG Trace

- Variable decelerations – repeated umbilical cord compression with each contraction resulting in fetal systemic hypertension mediated through baroreceptors.
- Late decelerations – ongoing utero-placental insufficiency mediated through chemoreceptors that respond to acidosis and increased carbon dioxide concentration.

Handbook of CTG Interpretation: From Patterns to Physiology, ed. Edwin Chandraharan. Published by Cambridge University Press. © Cambridge University Press 2017.

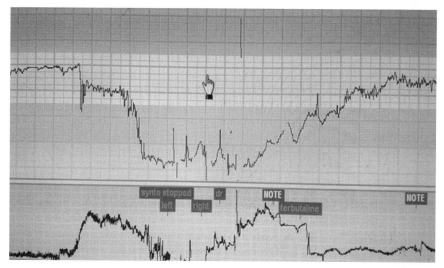

Figure 20.1 Uterine hypertonus after the administration of oxytocin, which is relieved after stopping oxytocin infusion and administration of terbutaline.

- Prolonged declarations – maternal hypotension, uterine hyperstimulation (hypertonus) often in response to oxytocin (Figure 20.1), sustained umbilical cord compression or cord prolapse.

Recommended Management

- *Oxygen*: High-flow oxygen administration via a non-rebreathe mask will increase maternal oxygen saturation and partial pressure, thus increasing fetal oxygenation. However, this is only recommended in patients with reduced maternal oxygen saturation level (e.g. maternal cardiac arrest or maternal hypovolumia secondary to massive placental abruption) as routine administration of oxygen may be even harmful due to vasoconstriction of the placental bed secondary to increased oxygen tension, especially in a growth-restricted fetus.
- *Fluid*: One litre rapid intravenous infusion (unless fluid restricted/contraindicated, i.e. preeclampsia), even if the woman is not hypovolemic, will improve venous return and cardiac output and, therefore, uterine blood flow. Fluid infusion may also help dilute oxytocin in cases of uterine hyperstimulation.
- *Maternal repositioning*: A change in maternal position, for example, left lateral, may relieve aortocaval compression and cardiac output.
- Stop oxytocics (i.e. syntocinon) and consider administration of tocolytics (e.g. terbutaline 0.25 mg subcutaneously) if there is evidence of hyperstimulation – this will improve utero-placental perfusion and reduce cord compression through uterine relaxation. Similarly, if prostaglandins are administered to induce labour, this must be removed immediately and tocolytics should be administered if there is no further improvement in the CTG trace.
- Vasopressors (e.g. adrenaline) if maternal hypotension occurs secondary to maternal collapse – this may be considered to restore cardiac output and maternal BP.

Key Tips to Optimize Outcome

- A combination of interventions may be of a greater benefit.
- Ensure continuous reassessment – after each intervention, it is important to observe for subsequent improvement in the CTG trace including a reduction in decelerations, a fall in baseline heart rate and improvement in baseline variability or, in cases of prolonged deceleration, recovery to normal baseline heart rate.
- Assess progress of labour and the 'wider clinical picture' after improvement in the CTG trace to determine whether continuation of labour is appropriate.
- In chronic hypoxia or umbilical cord prolapse, if a delay in delivery is anticipated (e.g. operating theatre being busy), tocolysis may help reduce hypoxic stress by abolishing uterine contractions until urgent delivery is accomplished.
- If atonic postpartum haemorrhage (PPH) is not responding to standard oxytocics after administration of terbutaline to relax the myometrium, propranolol 1 mg intravenously should be considered to reverse the effects of terbutaline after delivery in cases of refractory PPH not responding to standard oxytocic drugs.

Pitfalls

- Change in maternal position can, in some cases, result in worsening of cord compression; thus, further positions should be tried including the right lateral or knee-elbow position.
- Use of tocolysis to reduce uterine activity and to improve fetal condition may induce maternal tachycardia and hypotension (glyceryl trinitrate is not licenced as an acute tocolytic agent).
- A tocolytic may additionally predispose to atonic PPH during caesarean section if immediate delivery is accomplished.

Consequences of Mismanagement

- Worsening intrapartum hypoxic stress leading to hypoxic-ischaemic encephalopathy and perinatal death.
- Unnecessary operative interventions due to 'CTG abnormalities' secondary to uterine hyperstimulation, which is a correctable cause.

Exercise

1. A 29-year-old primigravida presented with spontaneous early labour at 39 + 4 weeks of gestation. She was commenced on oxytocin at 5 cm dilation for failure to progress. One hour later, her CTG trace (Figure 20.2) shows the following features.
   a. What is your diagnosis?

   Two hours later, the CTG trace shows the following features (Figure 20.3).

   b. What is your diagnosis?
   c. What action will you take?

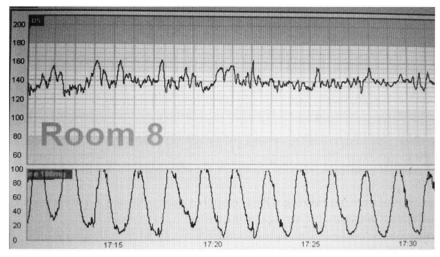

Figure 20.2

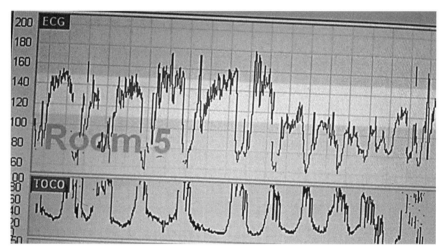

Figure 20.3

Further Reading

1. Kither, H. Monaghan, S. (2013) Intrauterine fetal resuscitation. *Anaesthesia and Intensive Care Medicine* 14 (7) 287–290.

2. Velayudhareddy, S. Kirankumar, H. (2010) Management of fetal asphyxia by intrauterine foetal resuscitation. *Indian Journal of Anaesthesia* 54 (5) 394–399.

3. Thurlow, JA. Kinsella, SM. (2002) Intrauterine resuscitation: active management of fetal distress. *International Journal of Obstetric Anaesthesia* 11, 105–116.

4. National Institute for Health and Clinical Excellence (2014) *Intrapartum Care CG190*. London: RCOG Press.

5. Tram, TS. Kulier, R. Hofmeyr, GJ. (2012) Acute tocolysis for uterine tachysystole or suspected fetal distress. *Cochrane Database of Systematic Reviews* 4.

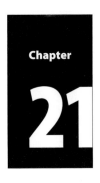

Chapter 21

Management of Prolonged Decelerations and Bradycardia

Rosemary Townsend and Edwin Chandraharan

Key Facts

- A prolonged deceleration indicates a need for urgent assessment and intervention to improve fetal oxygenation.
- Acute hypoxia caused by cord prolapse, placental abruption or uterine rupture mandates delivery without any delay.
- Most prolonged decelerations with an identifiable reversible cause will respond to conservative measures and recover within 9 minutes and do not require immediate delivery.
- Acute tocolysis is a useful treatment for prolonged deceleration secondary to uterine hyperstimulation.
- In the absence of an irreversible cause (placental abruption, umbilical cord prolapse and uterine rupture), the most important features of the CTG trace that predict the likelihood of recovery of an ongoing prolonged deceleration are baseline variability prior to the onset of deceleration and variability in the first 3 minutes of deceleration. In addition, if the fetal heart rate (FHR) is maintained >100 bpm during a prolonged deceleration, the likelihood of acidosis is low. Conversely, an acute drop in FHR <80 bpm may indicate acute intrapartum hypoxic insult and may lead to a rapid development of fetal acidosis if this persists for >3 minutes.

Management of Prolonged Decelerations

- A prolonged deceleration may be secondary to fetal hypoxia caused by reduced utero-placental perfusion or sustained cord compression. Nonhypoxic prolonged decelerations may also be seen during profound vagal stimulation, as is seen with increased intracranial pressure caused by head compression immediately before delivery of the head,[1] and not all prolonged decelerations are associated with the same degree of neonatal acidaemia.
- The outcome for the fetus will depend on the cause of deceleration, the fetal condition before deceleration and the preexisting placental reserves, and therefore, it is important to keep the whole clinical picture in mind.
- The fetal response to acute hypoxia is a chemoreflex response leading to prolonged deceleration and increased peripheral resistance.[2] The physiological aim is to reduce oxygenation of peripheral tissues to preserve cerebral and myocardial

Handbook of CTG Interpretation: From Patterns to Physiology, ed. Edwin Chandraharan. Published by Cambridge University Press. © Cambridge University Press 2017.

oxygenation (intense peripheral vasoconstriction) as well as to reduce myocardial workload (prolonged deceleration). Although these mechanisms exist to protect the central organs from hypoxic injury during an acute hypoxic or hypotensive insult, prolongation of deceleration may result in cardiac and neurological damage due to a reduction of perfusion pressure.

- Anaerobic metabolism takes place in vasoconstricted peripheral tissues with progressive lactic acid build-up and metabolic acidosis. In addition, carbon dioxide cannot be eliminated through the placenta during periods of reduced placental blood flow, causing a respiratory acidaemia. The respiratory component of acidaemia is rapidly eliminated when placental blood flow is restored, while metabolic acidosis takes longer to correct.

- Whereas, in the presence of subacute hypoxia, fetal pH levels fall at a rate of 0.01 per 2–3 minutes, during a period of acute hypoxia, fetal pH drops at a rate of 0.01 per minute. Increasing levels of fetal acidaemia will eventually lead to a disruption of cellular enzymes, tissue injury and death.

- With a significant reduction in heart rate, there must be a fall in cardiac output, whatever the cause, since the fetus does not have the capacity to increase stroke volume to compensate.[3] Peripheral vasoconstriction is an early response that enables the fetus to maintain near-normal levels of cerebral and myocardial blood flow in the early stages, but if the insult persists, these mechanisms will fail.

- The fetus prioritizes myocardial flow over cerebral blood flow, so the next CTG change to be observed will be reduced or absent variability as the fetal autonomic nervous system is compromised. As blood flow to the myocardium then fails, myocardial function will depend on glycogenolysis, and once the glycogen stores are depleted, the myocardium will also begin to fail.

- This period of time that will result in central organ decompensation will clearly be shorter in a growth-restricted fetus with lower glycogen stores.

- The presence of acute prolonged fall in heart rate requires rapid intervention from the care team. This does not mean that the response to every prolonged deceleration should be immediate delivery, and indeed the majority of prolonged decelerations will respond completely to simple conservative measures before either the brain or the myocardium is compromised.

- Having a well-practiced protocol for the management of prolonged decelerations will help avoid unnecessary interventions and distress for the patient while enabling the team to identify quickly those fetuses that will not respond to conservative measures.

Causes of Prolonged Decelerations

The first priority in the management of a prolonged deceleration is to establish the underlying cause as quickly as possible to facilitate appropriate management. To this end, it is useful to classify the causes as reversible and nonreversible (see Table 21.1).

Nonreversible Causes of Prolonged Decelerations

- There are three important nonreversible causes of acute hypoxia (prolonged decelerations) that require immediate delivery. Once a nonreversible cause is identified,

Table 21.1 Causes of prolonged decelerations

Reversible	Nonreversible
Hypotension	Placental abruption
Excessive uterine activity	Cord prolapse
Sustained umbilical cord compression	Uterine rupture

it is not appropriate to delay even 2 or 3 minutes to await recovery of the CTG, and delivery must be accomplished by the safest and most expeditious route.

- These three nonreversible events are cord prolapse, placental abruption and uterine rupture. In these situations, the compromise to fetal oxygenation is profound and cannot be reversed by any conservative measures (except in umbilical cord prolapse where acute tocolysis may relieve the compression of umbilical cord during uterine contractions). The immediate examination of the patient to identify these causes should occur simultaneously with intrauterine resuscitation measures (left lateral position, fluids, stopping oxytocin).

- Any assessment of the mother should start with the ABC (airway, breathing, circulation) approach and include action to correct any abnormality in maternal oxygenation or cardiovascular stability. Any condition that causes compromise to maternal oxygenation may also cause acute hypoxia in the fetus; however, the management of these conditions is out of the scope of this chapter. Maternal resuscitation takes priority and, in the context of a primarily maternal condition, should be all that is necessary to restore fetal oxygenation.

- Abdominal examination should take particular note of the tone of uterus, descent of fetal head or presence of fetal parts. A vaginal examination is necessary to rule out cord prolapse, to assess vaginal bleeding, receding presenting part and cervical dilatation should an emergency delivery be indicated.

- If any nonreversible cause of acute hypoxia is identified, delivery should be immediate, and this would usually be by caesarean section. Although, according to the NICE classification of urgency, a category 1 caesarean section should accomplish delivery <30 minutes in the setting of acute hypoxia with an irreversible cause, delivery after 15 minutes is associated with worsening fetal acidaemia and greater likelihood of admission to the neonatal unit.

Reversible Causes of Prolonged Decelerations

Maternal Hypotension

- Hypotension may occur in labour due to vagal stimulation, dehydration or peripheral vasodilatation associated with the administration of regional anaesthesia or a combination of all of these. In the assessment of a patient in the context of a prolonged deceleration, it is imperative to assess the blood pressure immediately and institute measures to correct hypotension.

- The supine position should be avoided for labouring women because of the association with aortocaval compression and associated reduced venous return and myocardial and placental perfusion.

Management of Hypotension

- Place the mother in left lateral position.
- Fluid resuscitation (in the setting of dehydration or acute hypotension after regional anaesthesia administration).

Excessive Uterine Activity (Tachysystole)

- Tachysystole is defined as excessive frequency of contractions with more than five contractions in 10 minutes for at least 20 minutes or averaged over 30 minutes. This will not always cause fetal hypoxia, and indeed many well-grown fetuses with adequate placental reserves will tolerate prolonged periods of tachysystole.
- Uterine hyperstimulation is the presence of CTG changes associated with tachysystole. In the event of CTG changes associated with prolonged hypertonic contractions or tachysystole, particularly during oxytocin administration, action should be taken to reduce the frequency and strength of uterine contractions.
- The first action should be to stop administration of any exogenous oxytocin (or removal of prostaglandins). In the presence of minor CTG changes – for example a rise in baseline or progressively longer decelerations with evidence of chemoreceptor activation – this may be sufficient.
- In severe acute or subacute hypoxia (including prolonged decelerations), acute tocolysis is often of benefit in rapidly restoring placental perfusion and reversing fetal hypoxia. Because tocolytics must be administered rapidly in the setting of a prolonged deceleration, it is recommended that the medication be stored in an easy-to-access area together with all the necessary equipment for administration. In our unit, a clearly marked emergency pack containing 250 µg terbutaline, a needle, syringe and cotton wool is centrally available and has been useful in reducing time to administration.
- Agents suitable for acute tocolysis include β-sympathomimetics such as terbutaline and ritodrine.[4] Because these drugs have been associated with maternal cardiac side effects when used for tocolysis for preterm labour, some alternatives have been trialled. There is some evidence that atosiban, a competitive oxytocin receptor antagonist that is commonly used in the treatment of preterm labour, may also be of benefit in acute tocolysis.[5,6] There is little evidence that magnesium sulphate has a role in acute tocolysis. Nitroglycerine may also be used, but is less effective than terbutaline and is more likely to provoke maternal hypotension.[7]
- There may be concern regarding the use of tocolytics immediately before delivery because the uterine relaxant effect could theoretically increase the risk of postpartum haemorrhage. While there is little evidence on the blood loss in deliveries where acute tocolysis has been used in labour for fetal compromise, in the case of tocolysis with terbutaline used to prolong pregnancies affected by placenta praevia, no significant difference in blood loss has been demonstrated.[8] In our clinical experience, no additional measures beyond routine oxytocics are required after delivery. If there is no response to oxytocics, 1 mg of propranolol may be administered to reverse the uterine relaxant effect of terbutaline.
- After the administration of an acute tocolytic, signs of improvement in the CTG may be anticipated within 2–5 minutes. This may simply be a return of normal variability and need not be a complete return to baseline. In certain circumstances, a second dose may

be appropriate. The team should remain on standby to perform an emergency delivery until it is clear that the CTG has normalized.

Management of Uterine Hyperstimulation

- Intrauterine resuscitation
- Stop oxytocin administration
- Acute tocolysis (e.g. with 250 µg subcutaneous terbutaline)

CTG Parameters That Predict Recovery of Prolonged Decelerations

- The majority of prolonged decelerations with a reversible cause will respond to conservative measures before delivery is indicated, and so the approach to the patient should be reassuring. The CTG features prior to and during deceleration are related to the chance of recovery, and familiarity with these features can help identify which patients really need to be transferred to the operating theatre and which can safely be managed in the delivery room.
- The preceding normal variability on the CTG trace is of importance because it may give information regarding the oxygenation of the fetus prior to the onset of current insult. In the case of a normal CTG with a stable baseline and normal variability, the risk of fetal hypoxia is low; therefore, it can be assumed that the fetus is starting from a normal acid–base balance. Conversely, if the preceding CTG showed evidence of fetal hypoxia with a rising baseline and reducing variability, it indicates that the fetus will not tolerate a long period of acute hypoxia.
- The variability on the CTG corresponds to the integrity of fetal autonomic nervous system, and in most cases variability is preserved in the first minutes of prolonged deceleration because cerebral oxygenation is maintained by the redistribution of cardiac output. If there is normal variability in the 3 minutes before deceleration and in the first 3 minutes of deceleration, then it is highly likely that the FHR will recover – 90 per cent in 6 minutes and 95 per cent in 9 minutes.
- Conversely, if there is reduced variability before prolonged deceleration, then even after recovery, as many as 44 per cent of fetuses may be compromised, and consideration should be given to delivery after consideration of the wider clinical picture.

Assessment of CTG Parameters

In a prolonged deceleration with a previously normal CTG and normal variability in the first 3 minutes of deceleration, recovery can safely be anticipated. In the presence of a preceding abnormal CTG, particularly with reduced variability, preparations for emergency delivery should be made.

When Should Delivery Occur?

- In the absence of nonreversible causes and after the institution of conservative measures for intrauterine resuscitation, the key clinical decision to be made is whether or not to initiate delivery, usually by caesarean section, unless the second stage of labour is well advanced and rapid instrumental delivery is possible.

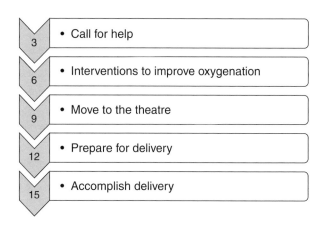

Figure 21.1 The '3,6,9,12,15' Rule.

- It is important to note that even moving the mother to the operating room and preparing for an emergency caesarean section should never preclude stepping down in the event of improvement in the CTG and that this should be communicated to the parents during the transfer process.
- The historical rule of thumb for timing of intervention has been the '3-6-9-12' rule (Figure 21.1). This has the advantage of being easily remembered in an emergency and encouraging timely transfer to theatre in the event of a severe prolonged deceleration; however, it does not encourage clinicians to consider the underlying cause of acute hypoxia.
- This can lead to overintervention in cases where the underlying cause could have been reversed, increased maternal risks from rushed procedures and unnecessary distress to mothers and partners. Failing to identify a cause of fetal hypoxia may also lead to a failure to prepare the team for massive blood loss associated with placental abruption or surgical complications associated with uterine rupture. In these nonreversible causes of acute hypoxia, even 3 minutes delay may lead to a difference in fetal condition at birth. It is important then to first identify the cause of prolonged deceleration so that the rule is not inappropriately applied.
- In the absence of a nonreversible cause of acute hypoxia, over 90 per cent of prolonged decelerations will recover by 6 minutes and 95 per cent within 9 minutes.[9] This observation is the foundation of the 3-6-9-12 rule. As has previously been discussed, in acute hypoxia it is expected that fetal pH will fall at a rate of 0.01 per minute. Therefore, a fetus starting with a pH of 7.3 and no other compromise would be expected to have a pH of 7.15 after 15 minutes and 7.0 after 30 minutes of continuous acute hypoxia.
- The CTG may well show signs of recovery at 6 minutes – an attempt to return to the baseline or an improvement in variability. In this case, with a normal preceding CTG and with no nonreversible causes of hypoxia, it would be reasonable to delay transfer to the operating room while continuing intrauterine resuscitation (e.g. Figure 21.1). In the event of a continuing prolonged deceleration, particularly with reducing variability, the 3-6-9-12 rule should be applied, allowing for reassessment and change of plan at every stage until operative delivery is actually commenced (Figure 21.2). In this situation, the possibility of concealed abruption, an occult cord prolapse or an undiagnosed scar dehiscence should be considered.

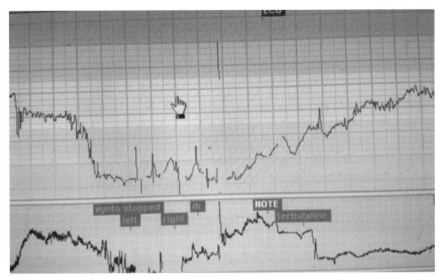

Figure 21.2 CTG showing normal baseline variability in 3 minutes before deceleration and in the first 3 minutes of deceleration. The repetitive prolonged contractions caused by syntocinon are the cause of deceleration, and at 6 minutes after syntocinon is stopped and terbutaline has been administered, the baseline starts to recover to normal and is fully recovered by 10 minutes. This patient was not transferred to theatre and the labour continued to a normal delivery.

After the Prolonged Deceleration Has Resolved

In most cases, it is appropriate to continue with the labour; however, the whole clinical picture should be carefully assessed before deciding to proceed. In the presence of ongoing hypoxic changes on the CTG, particularly in the context of chorioamnionitis or in the presence of meconium, it may be appropriate to consider delivery, especially if there are concerns regarding the progress of labour. In general, if the features observed on the CTG trace after recovery are similar to those seen before deceleration, it is appropriate to continue labour.

When Is It Safe to Restart Oxytocin?

It is often the case that tachysystole occurs as the endogenous production of and sensitivity to oxytocin increases as labour progresses and there may be no need to restart exogenous oxytocin infusions. If augmentation with oxytocin is necessary in order to continue the labour, there should be clear evidence of fetal well-being in the form of normal variability and a stable baseline before restarting an oxytocin infusion, and it should be restarted at a lower infusion rate than that being used previously.

Suggested Approach to Management of Prolonged Decelerations

1. Assess the patient for nonreversible causes while commencing conservative measures. (If found deliver immediately)
2. Assess the CTG for features that predict recovery

3. Treat reversible causes – consider fluid administration, stop oxytocin and consider acute tocolysis
4. Reassess the CTG and clinical picture

Management of Prolonged Decelerations

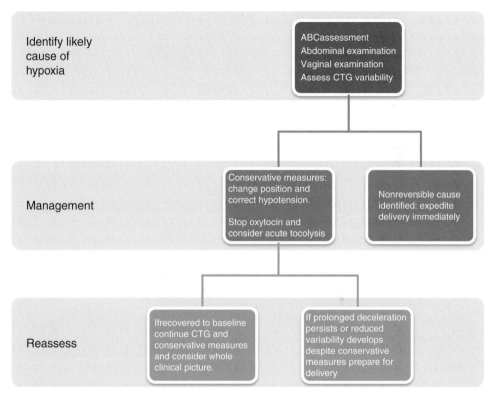

Identify likely cause of hypoxia	ABCassessment Abdominal examination Vaginal examination Assess CTG variability
Management	Conservative measures: change position and correct hypotension. Stop oxytocin and consider acute tocolysis	Nonreversible cause identified: expedite delivery immediately
Reassess	Ifrecovered to baseline continue CTG and conservative measures and consider whole clinical picture.	If prolonged deceleration persists or reduced variability develops despite conservative measures prepare for delivery

Figure 21.3

Management of Fetal Bradycardia

A fetal bradycardia is a baseline value <110 bpm for >10 minutes. This could occur in the setting of acute hypoxia that lasts for >10 minutes, in which case the onset would be sudden and a cause would usually be identifiable and management would be as described earlier. There are many other causes of a sustained baseline heart rate <110 bpm and careful consideration of these causes should be made if the CTG pattern is not in keeping with an acute deceleration.

A FHR of 100–110 bpm may be normal, particularly in a postdates fetus. In this case variability will be normal, accelerations are likely to be present and the baseline is likely to be consistent with previous fetal heart measurements. No further intervention is required and in fact if no other risk factors exist this is not an indication for continuous EFM in labour.

Other causes for fetal bradycardia include placental transfer of maternal medications, particularly beta-adrenoceptor blockers.[10] Beta-blockers depress the activity of the sympathetic nervous system that would normally tend to increase the FHR. They may also be associated with a reduction in variability, however it would be expected that the variability would not be entirely absent (often described as 'pencil tip') and accelerations, while reduced in amplitude, would be expected to be present.

Fetal arrhythmias, particularly complete heart block, may appear on CTG as a profound bradycardia. Congenital heart block is associated with a significant risk of mortality but is rare, and the detailed management is out of the scope of this chapter. The bradycardia in this case does not represent acute compromise, however over time the lowered cardiac output and volume overload may cause myocardial damage, dilated cardiomyopathy and impaired ventricular systolic function.[11] The worst outcomes are seen with rates <50–55 bpm.[12] Diagnosis and delivery planning require assessment by a fetal medicine specialist.

Common Pitfalls

Failure to identify underlying cause of prolonged deceleration/bradycardia is the most common mistake made. As highlighted above, this may lead to inappropriate intervention, including major surgery on the mother and equally may lead to a lack of preparation for serious obstetric emergencies.

Failure to use acute tocolysis when uterine hyperstimulation is the cause of fetal hypoxia. In uterine hyperstimulation, one may well do a caesarean section and deliver a baby with a cord pH of 7.01 and then may congratulate the team on a disaster averted. Instead, an obstetrician should aim to be able to congratulate himself/herself on achieving a normal delivery with normal gases and maintaining one's own blood pressure in the normal range by a simple administration of terbutaline (to the mother) to treat uterine hyperstimulation so as to continue labour.

Failure to reassess the situation. Failure to stop a caesarean section when the CTG has become reassuring is common and may lead to entirely unnecessary surgery with significant consequences for the mother. Additionally, the fetus that is delivered only minutes after recovering from a significant period of hypoxia is likely to be in worse condition at birth than one with time to recover. Equally, clinging to the hope that the CTG will recover after 10 minutes when there are no signs of improvement is an unnecessary and dangerous delay for the fetus.

Exercise

1. A primigravida is induced at 41 + 5 weeks of gestation for postdates after a normal pregnancy. The CTG up to this point has been entirely normal with a baseline rate of 130 bpm and variability of 5–15 bpm. At 11:49, a deceleration begins and the attending midwife appropriately moves the mother into the left lateral position.
   You are called to the room at 11:54.
   a. What are the first steps you would take to assess the patient?
   b. What is the likely cause of this prolonged deceleration?
   c. What would your management be?
   d. What features on the CTG are reassuring?
   e. What features on the CTG are concerning?
   Now consider the trace again (Figure 21.5).

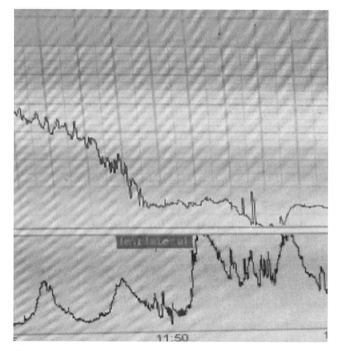

Figure 21.4

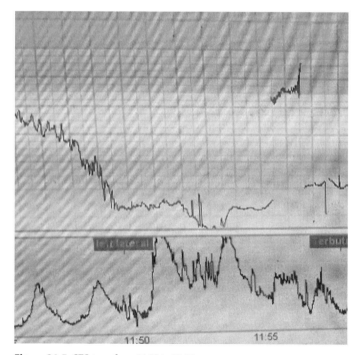

Figure 21.5 CTG trace from 11:55 to 11:56.

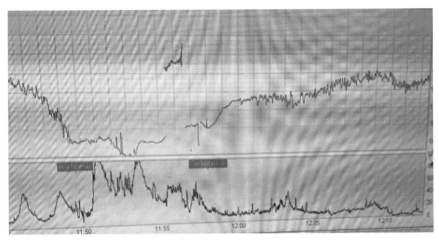

Figure 21.6 CTG trace after administration of terbutaline.

f.   What phenomenon is demonstrated at 11:55–11:56?

g.   Terbutaline is administered at 11:57. At 11:58 what would your next action be?

Figure 21.6 shows the full trace indicating first recovery of the baseline and second restoration of normal variability suggesting an intact neurological system. The tocograph clearly demonstrates that the uterine activity has been temporarily abolished.

h.   What might you expect to see next on the CTG?

References

1.   Mocsáry P, Gaál J, Komáromy B, Mihály G, Pohánka O, Surányi S. Relationship between fetal intracranial pressure and fetal heart rate during labor. *Am J Obstet Gynecol*. Elsevier; 1970 Jan 2;106(3):407–11.

2.   Giussani DA, Spencer JA, Moore PJ, Bennet L, Hanson MA. Afferent and efferent components of the cardiovascular reflex responses to acute hypoxia in term fetal sheep. *J Physiol*. 1993 Feb;461:431–49.

3.   Thornburg KL, Morton MJ. Filling and arterial pressures as determinants of left ventricular stroke volume in fetal lambs. *Am J Physiol Hear Circ Physiol*. 1986 Nov 1;251(5):H961–8.

4.   Chandraharan E, Arulkumaran S. Acute tocolysis. *Curr Opin Obstet Gynecol*. 2005 Apr;17(2):151–6.

5.   Afschar P, Schöll W, Bader A, Bauer M, Winter R. A prospective randomised trial of atosiban versus hexoprenaline for acute tocolysis and intrauterine resuscitation. *BJOG*. 2004 Apr;111(4):316–8.

6.   de Heus R, Mulder EJH, Derks JB, Kurver PHJ, van Wolfswinkel L, Visser GHA. A prospective randomized trial of acute tocolysis in term labour with atosiban or ritodrine. *Eur J Obstet Gynecol Reprod Biol*. 2008 Aug;139(2):139–45.

7.   Pullen KM, Riley ET, Waller SA, Taylor L, Caughey AB, Druzin ML, et al. Randomized comparison of intravenous terbutaline vs nitroglycerin for acute intrapartum fetal resuscitation. *Am J Obstet Gynecol*. 2007 Oct;197(4):414.e1–6.

8.   Besinger RE, Moniak CW, Paskiewicz LS, Fisher SG, Tomich PG. The effect of tocolytic use in the management of symptomatic placenta previa. *Am J Obstet Gynecol*. 1995 Jun;172(6):1770–5; discussion 1775–8.

9.   Chandraharan E, Arulkumaran S. Prevention of birth asphyxia: responding

appropriately to cardiotocograph (CTG) traces. *Best Pract Res Clin Obstet Gynaecol.* Elsevier; 2007 Aug 8;21(4):609–24.

10. Boutroy MJ. Fetal and neonatal effects of the beta-adrenoceptor blocking agents. *Dev Pharmacol Ther.* 1987 Jan;10(3):224–31.

11. Donofrio MT, Gullquist SD, Mehta ID, Moskowitz WB. Congenital complete heart block: fetal management protocol, review of the literature, and report of the smallest successful pacemaker implantation. *J Perinatol.* 2004 Jan 22;24(2):112–7.

12. Jaeggi ET, Hamilton RM, Silverman ED, Zamora SA, Hornberger LK. Outcome of children with fetal, neonatal or childhood diagnosis of isolated congenital atrioventricular block. A single institution's experience of 30 years. *J Am Coll Cardiol.* 2002 Jan 2;39(1):130–7.

13. Gull I, Jaffa AJ, Oren M, Grisaru D, Peyser MR, Lessing JB. Acid accumulation during end-stage bradycardia in term fetuses: how long is too long? *Br J Obstet Gynaecol.* 1996 Nov;103(11):1096–101.

14. WILLIAMS K. Fetal heart rate parameters predictive of neonatal outcome in the presence of a prolonged deceleration. *Obstet Gynecol.* 2002 Nov;100(5):951–4.

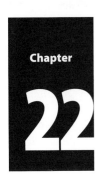

Chapter

22

ST-Analyser (STAN)
Principles and Physiology

Ana Piñas Carrillo and Edwin Chandraharan

Key Facts

- A recent systematic review of randomized controlled trials has concluded that the use of STAN reduced the incidence of use of fetal blood sampling and metabolic acidosis.
- STAN has been shown to reduce the interobserver variation when indicating interventions in the presence of intermediate or abnormal CTG traces.
- The principle of STAN is to assess the oxygenation of a central organ (the fetal heart). It helps to differentiate between a fetus that is exposed to hypoxic stress but compensating well and maintaining a good oxygenation in the myocardium from the fetus that switches to anaerobic metabolism in the myocardium and depends on catecholamine-mediated glycogenolysis to respond to negative energy balance in the myocardium.
- The fetal ECG is monitored through a fetal scalp electrode. As soon as it is applied, the STAN machine calculates (over 4–5 minutes) the normal T/QRS ratio for that particular fetus and establishes it as the 'baseline value'. From this moment, the machine analyses every 30 ECG complexes (i.e. if baseline fetal heart rate (FHR) is 150 bpm, there would be five analyses in 1 minute) and compares them with the original 'baseline value'. Each of them is recorded on the CTG trace as a cross ('X'). When the analysed ECG complexes differ significantly from 'baseline value', it will be flagged up as an 'ST event'.
- In the presence of an 'ST event', it is necessary to classify the CTG trace according to STAN guidelines (normal, intermediate or abnormal) first and then to determine if the 'ST event' is significant and requires any action. Conversely, if the ST event is not significant, no further action is required at this time.

Key Features on the STAN

Please see Figure 22.1.
- There are three types of 'ST events': episodic T/QRS rise, baseline T/QRS rise and biphasic events.
- 'Episodic T/QRS rise' event appears when the T/QRS ratio rises in response to a short-lasting hypoxia for <10 minutes. The significance depends on the magnitude of rise and classification of the CTG trace. If the CTG trace is classified as normal, the ST event is not significant as it can be secondary to fetal movements and resultant release of

---

Handbook of CTG Interpretation: From Patterns to Physiology, ed. Edwin Chandraharan. Published by Cambridge University Press. © Cambridge University Press 2017.

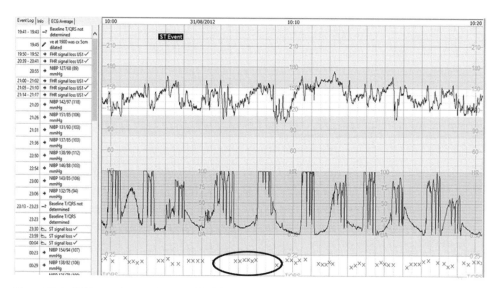

Figure 22.1 STAN trace showing ST event (black box), event log (left-hand column) and crosses ('x') – each 'x' (oval) represents 30 fetal ECG complexes.

catecholamine-mediated myocardial glycogenolysis; if the CTG trace is intermediate, a greater increase in the T/QRS ratio is allowed before it becomes significant than if the CTG trace is classified as abnormal.

- 'Baseline T/QRS rise' indicates a longer-lasting hypoxia (>10 minutes) with the resultant increase in the T/QRS ratio persisting for >10 minutes. The magnitude of rise is shown on the screen (event log), and the significance depends again on magnitude and classification of the CTG trace.

- 'Biphasic ST' appears when there is a shift in the ST segment. There are three degrees of biphasic ST events (grades 1–3). Repetitive grade 2 and 3 biphasic events are significant in the presence of an intermediate or abnormal trace as they may reflect instability of the myocardial membrane secondary to hypoxia and resultant changes in the morphology of ST segment of the fetal ECG complex.

- Event log indicates documentation by clinicians (e.g. vaginal examination, blood pressure monitoring, administration of oxytocin) as well as by the computer (e.g. type and magnitude of ST events, loss of contact).

Key Pathophysiology behind Patterns Seen on the CTG Trace

- The fetal ECG reflects the oxygenation of a central organ, the myocardium, which is the last organ to fail when a fetus is exposed to hypoxia.
- *Physiology behind 'T/QRS ST events'*: The fetus releases catecholamines (emergency hormone) that increase the FHR and also activate 'glycogenolysis' in the myocardium to increase the glucose available for the heart to function. The process of 'glycogenolysis' results in a release of potassium ions which have been stored within glycogen, and the resultant 'hyperkalemia' produces a rise in 'T waves' and an increase on 'T/QRS ratio'. This phenomenon results in 'T/QRS ST events'.

- *Physiology behind 'biphasic ST events'*: The ST segment reflects the refractory period (isoelectric) after depolarization (myocardial contraction) and before repolarization when there is no transfer of ions through the myocardial cells. In the presence of a disturbance to the myocardial pump function (secondary to hypoxia, infection, prematurity or cardiac defects), the ST segment shifts upwards or downwards resulting on a biphasic 'ST event', reflecting myocardial membrane dysfunction.

Recommended Management

- In the presence of a normal CTG trace, any 'ST events' can be managed with expectant management, as they are not significant at this stage. Most commonly, they are secondary to fetal movements that also release catecholamines.
- In the presence of a preterminal trace, delivery should be expedited regardless of the presence or absence of 'ST events'.
- In the presence of a significant ST event during the first or passive second stage of labour, interventions to improve utero-placental oxygenation need to be instituted. These include stopping oxytocin infusion, administration of intravenous fluids, postural changes and/or acute tocolysis (terbutaline) to improve fetal oxygenation. If the changes observed on the CTG improve and/or there are no further ST events, labour can be allowed to continue. If there are further significant ST events, CTG should be reclassified, and if the ST-events are significant and if no further conservative measures are possible, then immediate delivery (within 20 minutes) is indicated.
- During active second stage of labour, any *significant* ST event should be managed with immediate operative delivery (by the safest and quickest mode of birth) as soon as possible unless spontaneous vaginal delivery is expected in the following 5 to 10 minutes.
- CTG changes and ST events should always be correlated with the clinical picture (presence of meconium, chorioamnionitis, vaginal bleeding, growth restriction). Immediate delivery may be indicated in the presence of any of these risk factors regardless of the significance of ST events.

Key Tips to Optimize Outcome

- Remember STAN can only be used in fetuses >36 weeks of gestational age as the endocardial–epicardial interphase may be underdeveloped and interfere with signal conduction leading to multiple ST events (most commonly biphasic ST events). For the same reason, it cannot be used in fetuses with structural cardiac defects.
- In the presence of infection, any ST event, even in the presence of an intermediary trace, may be regarded as significant.
- If, when applying the fetal scalp electrode, repetitive ST events appear, ensure that fetal presentation is cephalic. If the fetus is presenting by breech, ECG complexes will be inverted and the machine interprets this as repeated biphasic ST events due to perceived inversion of ST-segment of the fetal ECG complex (i.e. will be recorded as a negative wave). If a decision is made to continue labour in anticipation of an assisted vaginal breech delivery, then the STAN machine has a 'breech mode' to invert the ECG complex so that biphasic events can be stopped and the fetus can be continuously monitored using the STAN technology.

Common Pitfalls

- Relying on STAN in the presence of chorioamnionitis. The STAN is a test of hypoxia and not for infection. In the presence of an infection, there may not be any ST events until the very final stages when the infection is affecting the oxygenation to central organs (i.e. fetal myocardium leading to myocarditis).
- Chorioamnionitis may lead to repeated biphasic ST events due to the inflammatory damage to myocardial membrane. In this case, the CTG may not show significant decelerations, and a high index of clinical suspicion of ongoing chorioamnionitis should be exercised and labour should be managed accordingly.
- Applying the STAN in the absence of a stable baseline heart rate and a reassuring variability. The STAN device calculates the normal ECG complex for each fetus during the first 4–5 minutes. It is not possible to rely on STAN when it is applied during ongoing subacute hypoxia with a loss of a stable baseline and/or reassuring variability
- Erroneous monitoring of the maternal heart rate (MHR) as FHR. When MHR is being monitored, the P-waves would be absent on the ECG complexes as the signal (maternal P-wave) is not powerful enough to be transmitted to the fetal scalp electrode.
- Unnecessary interventions for a normal CTG trace when ST events are flagged up or lack of intervention on a preterminal trace in the absence of ST events.

Consequences of Mismanagement

- Unnecessary interventions (operative delivery) due to nonadherence to STAN guidelines
- Stillbirth
- Neonatal death
- Hypoxic-ischaemic encephalopathy and subsequent cerebral palsy
- Neonatal sepsis – when relying on STAN and ignoring signs of ongoing clinical chorioamnionitis

Recent Developments

- A large multicentre randomized controlled trial from the United States of America in 2015 reported that the use of STAN did not reduce operative delivery rates.[7] However, the limitation of this study, including the incorrect classification system which has been used in the study group has been highlighted in a recent editorial.[8] A recent meta-analysis of six randomized controlled trials on STAN comprising of 26446 women, including the US Trial, has still concluded that the use of STAN is associated with a 36% reduction in metabolic acidosis, which was statistically significant.[9] In addition, there was a statistically significant reduction in operative vaginal delivery rate as well as the rate of fetal scalp blood sampling.

Therefore, in the authors' opinion based on published systematic evidence, compared to other adjunctive tests (i.e. pulse oximetry, fetal scalp pH and lactate), which have been shown to have no robust scientific evidence of benefit, STAN is the only adjunctive test which has been shown to be beneficial in 2016 (i.e. a statistically significant reduction in metabolic acidosois, fetal blood sampling and operative vaginal births). However, training in fetal physiology prior to introducing STAN is essential to maximize its benefits and to minimize harm.

Further Reading

1. Chandraharan E. STAN: an introduction to its use, limitations and caveats. *Obs Gyn Midwifery Prod News.* 2010. Sep 2: 18-22.

2. Neilson JP. Fetal electrocardiogram (ECG) for fetal monitoring during labour. *Cochrane Database Syst Rev.* 2006;3: Art. No.: CD000116. DOI:10.1002/14651858. CD000116.pub2.

3. Amer-Wåhlin I, Hellsten C, Norén H, Hagberg H, Herbst A, Kjellmer I, Lilja H, Lindoff C, Månsson M, Mårtensson L, Olofsson P, Sundström AK, Marál K. Cardiotocography only versus cardiotocography plus ST analysis of fetal electrocardiogram for intrapartum fetal monitoring: a Swedish randomised controlled trial. *Lancet.* 2001;358:534–8.

4. Antonia C, Ayres-de-Campos D, Fernanda C, Cristina S, Joao B. Prediction of neonatal acidemia by computer analysis of fetal heart rate and ST event signals. *Am J Obstet Gynecol.* 2009;201:464e1–6.

5. Westerhuis ME, van Horen E, Kwee A, van der Tweel I, Visser GH, Moons KG. Inter- and intra-observer agreement of intrapartum ST analysis of the fetal electrocardiogram in women monitored by STAN. *BJOG.* 2009;116(4):545–51.

6. Olofsson P, Ayres-de-Campos D, Kessler J, Tendal B, Yli BM, Devoe L. A critical appraisal of the evidence for using cardiotocography plus ECG ST interval analysis for fetal surveillance in labor. Part II: the meta-analyses. *Acta Obstet Gynecol Scand.* 2014;93(6):571–86.

7. Belfort MA, Saade GR, Thom E, Blackwell SC, Reddy UM, Thorp JM Jr, et al. A Randomized Trial of Intrapartum Fetal ECG ST-Segment Analysis. *N Engl J Med.* 2015;373:632–41.

8. Bhide A, Chandraharan E, Acharya G. Fetal monitoring in labor: Implications of evidence generated by new systematic review. *Acta Obstet Gynecol Scand.* 2016 Jan;95(1):5–8.

9. Blix E, Brurberg KG, Reierth E, Reinar LM, Øian P. STwaveform analysis vs. cardiotocography alone for intrapartum fetal monitoring: A systematic review and meta-analysis of randomized trials. *Acta Obstet Gynecol Scand.* 2015;95:16–27.

ST-Analyser

Case Examples and Pitfalls

Ana Piñas Carrillo and Edwin Chandraharan

Key Principles

- ST-Analyser (STAN) is only validated for monitoring fetuses >36 + 0 weeks of gestation and should not be used in fetuses <35 weeks + 6 days of gestation.
- Contraindications to the application of fetal scalp electrode (e.g. any maternal infection with increased risk of vertical transmission through a defect in the fetal skin and fetal haemorrhagic disorders which may increase the risk of scalp haemorrhage) should be excluded.
- Fetus should retain the capacity to respond to evolving intrapartum hypoxic stress (i.e. should have a stable baseline fetal heart rate (FHR) and a reassuring variability indicative of good oxygenation of the central organs).
- STAN should not be commenced in the presence of an unstable baseline FHR (i.e. myocardial hypoxia), reduced baseline variability with preceding decelerations (hypoxia to the central nervous system) or in the presence of a preterminal trace indicative of total loss of the ability to respond to hypoxia.
- STAN is a test to detect intrapartum hypoxia. However, other pathways of fetal neurological damage (e.g. meconium aspiration syndrome, chorioamnionitis and inflammatory brain damage) should be considered while using STAN.
- CTG should be classified (Table 23.1) and STAN guidelines (Table 23.2) should be used while using STAN in clinical practice. Algorithms such as the '6C' approach (Figure 23.1) may aid in management.

Case 1. Commencement of STAN

The CTG trace shows a stable baseline FHR and a reassuring baseline variability prior to commencement of STAN. Appearance of 'crosses' or 'x' below the tocograph indicates that the analysis of fetal ECG has commenced (Figure 23.2). The 'event log' indicates that the 'baseline T/QRS was determined at 18:36 hours'. Therefore, it is appropriate to rely on STAN from this time onwards.

Each 'x' represents an average of 30 ECG complexes, and therefore, 4 'x's are seen in a box (1 minute) because baseline FHR is 140 bpm ($30 \times 4 = 120$).

STAN requires approximately 120 'x's (i.e. approximately 4 minutes if baseline FHR is 120 bpm) to calculate a baseline T/QRS ratio for an individual fetus. Subsequently, it compares the average of 30 ECG complexes with this original baseline T/QRS ratio as well as the

Handbook of CTG Interpretation: From Patterns to Physiology, ed. Edwin Chandraharan. Published by Cambridge University Press. © Cambridge University Press 2017.

Table 23.1 STAN guidelines: classification of the CTG trace

Cardiotocographic classification	Baseline heart frequency	Variability reactivity	Decelerations
Normal	110–150 bpm	5–25 bpm accelerations	Early decelerations Uncomplicated variable decelerations with a duration of <60 seconds and a beat loss of <60 bpm
Intermediary*	100–110 bpm 150–170 bpm Short bradycardia episode	>25 bpm without accelerations <5 bpm for >40 min	Uncomplicated variable decelerations with a duration of <60 seconds and a beat loss of >60 bpm
Abnormal	150–170 bpm and reduced variability >170 bpm	<5 bpm for >60 minutes Sinusoidal pattern	Repeated late decelerations Complicated variable decelerations with a duration of >60 seconds
Preterminal	Total lack of variability and reactivity with or without decelerations or bradycardia		

*Combination of several intermediary observations will result in an abnormal CTG.

Table 23.2 STAN guidelines: interpretation of ST events

ST events	Episodic T/QRS rise	Baseline T/QRS rise	Biphasic ST
Normal CTG	Expectant management and continued observation		
Intermediary CTG	>0.15	>0.10	3 biphasic log messages
Abnormal CTG	>0.10	>0.05	2 biphasic log messages
Preterminal CTG	Immediate delivery		

ST segment of the fetal ECG to determine whether there is a significant change in the T/QRS ratio or the ST Segment.

In addition, to ensure adequate ECG signals, crosses ('x') should not be absent continuously for >4 minutes and there should be a minimum of 10 'x's in any 10-minute period.

Case 2. STAN Events on a Normal CTG Trace

Repeated fetal movements can result in fetal catecholamine surge as a part of 'startle response' leading to glycogenolysis in the myocardium to release extra energy. This results in the release of potassium ions stored within glycogen into the myocardial cells as glycogen is broken down to glucose to provide extra energy substrate for the myocardial cell. Increased intracellular myocardial potassium level leads to tall 'T' waves on the ECG complexes and the generation of ST event (Figure 23.3).

Such false-positive ST events are common with repeated fetal movements, especially if there is a confluence of accelerations (Figure 23.3). No intervention is required as the CTG trace is entirely normal with no evidence of ongoing hypoxia (Table 23.2).

Check
- Gestational Age > 36 +0 weeks
- No Contraindications for FSE (e.g. infections)
- Not in active second stage of labour with an abnormal trace
- Absence of Acute intrapartum accidents, sinusoidal pattern or chronic hypoxia
- Fetus has a stable baseline fetal heart rate and reassuring variability

Consider Wider Clinical Picture
- Thick Meconium staining of amniotic fluid
- Clinical or subclinical chorioamnionitis
- Presence of a uterine scar – uterine rupture is unpredictable
- Evidence of feto-maternal haemorrhage (Atypical Sinusoidal Pattern)
- Failure to progress in labour
- Fetal Cardiac Malformations

Classify CTG
- Normal
- Intermediary or Abnormal but the fetus has a stable baseline fetal heart rate and reassuring variability

If the CTG is Preterminal, an immediate delivery is required

ST Events Whilst Monitoring

Correlate Type and Magnitude of ST Events with the CTG Trace
- Episodic T/QRS (>0.05 or > 0.10)
- Baseline T/QRS (>0.10 or > 0.15)
- Biphasic Events (2 or 3 Messages)
- Non-Significant ST Event – continue observation
- Significant – Immediate Corrective Action

Corrective Action
- Stop Oxytocin infusion
- Change Maternal Position
- Administer intravenous fluids
- Consider Tocolysis if appropriate
- Stop maternal active pushing if evidence of subacute hypoxia

Cascade
Immediate Delivery in cases of
- Preterminal CTG Traces
- Acute intrapartum Accidents (Abruption, Umbilical Cord Prolapse, acute feto-maternal haemorrhage or Uterine Rupture)
- Failure of conservative measures to correct abnormalities on the CTG Trace
- Significant ST Events in Active second stage of labour

Figure 23.1 Suggested algorithm: 6C approach for use of STAN in clinical practice.

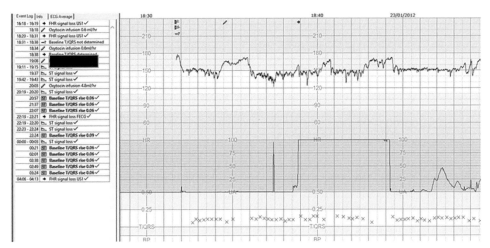

Figure 23.2 Stable baseline and reassuring baseline variability at the commencement of STAN monitoring. Note the event log.

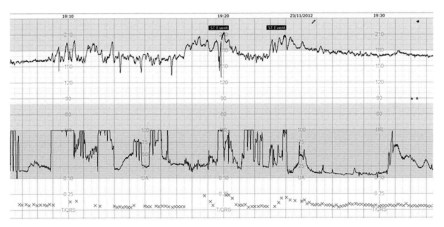

Figure 23.3 'Episodic' ST events secondary to repeated fetal movements. Note the abrupt increase in 'x's coinciding with the ST events confirming that there was an abrupt increase in the height of 'T' wave of fetal ECG due to intracellular release of potassium secondary to catecholamine-mediated glycogenolysis.

Case 3. Nonsignificant 'Episodic' STAN Events

Even if the STAN generates ST events, no action is needed if the magnitude of the event does not meet the threshold for intervention (Table 23.2). Therefore, every ST event that is noted on the monitor does not require an intervention.

The onset of maternal active pushing may result in the development of hypoxia within 10 minutes, leading to the generation of an ST event (Figure 23.4). However, even if the magnitude of episodic T/QRS event is 0.10, if the CTG trace is not abnormal, no intervention is required. In an intermediary CTG, a higher threshold (>0.15) would be required to warrant an intervention (Table 23.2).

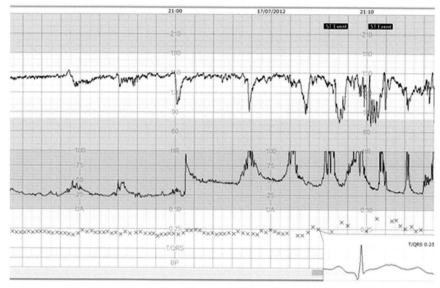

Figure 23.4 Worsening decelerations with the onset of maternal active pushing and transient increase in the 'x' in response to the release of intracellular potassium ions secondary to catecholamine-mediated myocardial glycogenolysis. The ECG complex also shows an elevation of the ST segment. However, no intervention is required as the type and magnitude of ST event is not significant for the observed CTG changes.

Case 4. Abnormal CTG without Significant ST Events

If the CTG remains abnormal despite absence of any significant ST events, a careful assessment should be made to ensure that the signal quality is adequate. In the presence of meconium staining of amniotic fluid and/or ongoing infection (i.e. chorioamnionitis), coexisting hypoxia can significantly worsen perinatal outcomes. Therefore, in the presence of deep prolonged decelerations and baseline tachycardia (Figure 23.5) and/or loss of baseline FHR variability, asphyxia-mediated intrapartum meconium aspiration syndrome and fetal inflammatory brain damage may occur, despite the absence of ST events.

Clinicians should appreciate the fact that STAN is a test of hypoxia and would not predict or diagnose meconium aspiration syndrome or diagnose ongoing inflammatory brain damage secondary to clinical or subclinical chorioamnionitis. Therefore, management decisions should be made based on the degree of CTG abnormalities noted, parity, cervical dilatation, progress of labour, need for augmentation with oxytocin and fetal reserve.

If other risk factors are absent and the CTG is abnormal, it is appropriate to continue labour in the absence of ST events, and conservative measures such as changing maternal position to avoid umbilical cord compression may be attempted to improve the CTG. However, in the presence of other risk factors such as thick meconium staining of amniotic fluid or clinical chorioamnionitis, intrapartum management should not depend on the absence of significant ST event alone. It is recommended that in the presence of clinical chorioamnionitis, an intermediary CTG should be upgraded to an abnormal CTG while interpreting ST events to recognize the fact that coexisting inflammation lowers the threshold at which hypoxia can damage the brain cells.

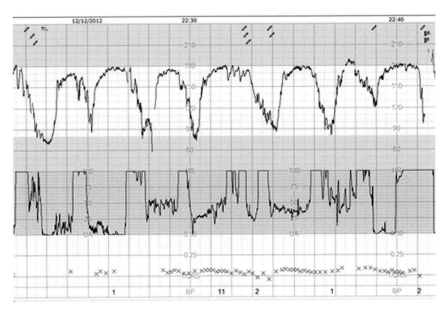

Figure 23.5 Ongoing complicated (or atypical) variable decelerations and increasing baseline FHR secondary to evolving hypoxia. Although the CTG is 'abnormal' according to STAN guidelines, there are no ST events and the signal quality is good ('x's are absent only for 2 minutes).

Case 5. Abnormal CTG with a Significant STAN Events

Any significant ST event requires an immediate intervention to improve utero-placental circulation (changing maternal position, stopping oxytocin infusion with or without administration of tocolytics and/or administration of intravenous fluids,) and if this is not possible, an urgent delivery should be accomplished within 20 minutes of the significant ST event. This holds true during first stage of labour and passive second stage of labour. A significant ST event on an abnormal CTG (Figure 23.6) requires an urgent intervention. The 'event log' would highlight the type and magnitude of the ST event (Figure 23.6).

During active second stage of labour (i.e. after the onset of active maternal pushing), immediate operative delivery (within 20 minutes) should be carried out, unless a spontaneous vaginal delivery is imminent within the next 10 minutes. This is because the evolution of hypoxia could be very rapid during active second stage of labour. If a delay in delivery is anticipated, maternal pushing should be stopped to rapidly improve fetal oxygenation.

If CTG has improved with conservative measures, it is appropriate to continue labour with close observation. If there are repeated ST events, the timing of the very first ST event should be considered in formulating a management plan. Worsening magnitude of ST events (e.g. baseline T/QRS ratios of 0.06, 0.09, 0.11, etc.) over time would indicate a progressively worsening hypoxic insult to the fetus, and urgent action should be taken to improve uteroplacental oxygenation, and if this is not possible or appropriate (e.g. placental abruption or uterine rupture), an immediate operative delivery should be undertaken.

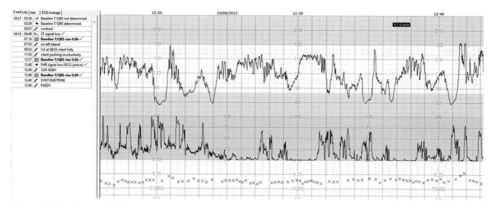

Figure 23.6 Abnormal CTG trace with repeated complicated (or atypical) variable decelerations lasting >60 seconds. The event log highlights baseline T/QRS ratio of 0.06, which is significant for an abnormal CTG according to STAN guidelines.

Pitfalls with the Use of STAN

Human error with regard to CTG interpretation and appropriate classification remains the main concern. In addition, failure to incorporate the wider clinical picture such as presence of thick meconium staining of amniotic fluid or evidence of clinical chorioamnionitis also may lead to poor outcomes.

Failure to adhere to STAN guidelines (commencing STAN monitoring in preterm fetuses or fetuses with known cardiac malformations), failure to accomplish delivery within 20 minutes in the presence of a significant ST event or commencement of STAN monitoring in the presence of preterminal CTG or chronic hypoxia (i.e. loss of baseline FHR variability) may also lead to poor outcomes.

Conclusions

STAN determines oxygenation of the fetal myocardium and the capacity of the myocardium to deal with ongoing hypoxic stress via the onset of anaerobic metabolism, catecholamine-mediated cardiac glycogenolysis and consequent release of potassium ions within the myocardial cell. If the T/QRS ratio is significantly higher than the ratio calculated within the first 4 minutes of commencement of STAN monitoring, an ST event will be generated.

Intervention should be based on the type and magnitude of ST event as well as the classification of the CTG. Additional risk factors such as the presence of meconium staining of amniotic fluid, evidence of ongoing chorioamnionitis, lack of progress of labour, reduced physiological reserve of the fetus etc., should also be considered, and one should not merely rely on STAN alone.

It should be noted that if a fetus has exhausted all its reserves and does not have the capacity to mount a compensatory response to ongoing hypoxic stress (i.e. preterminal CTG trace), ST events may not be seen. This is because of depletion of myocardial energy stores (i.e. glycogen) and the resultant absence of catecholamine-mediated glycogenolysis and consequent absence of any further changes in ST segment or T/QRS ratio.

Further Reading

1. Chandraharan E. STAN: an introduction
    to its use, limitations and caveats. *Obs Gyn
    Midwifery Prod News*; 2010.

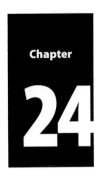

Chapter

Role of a Computerized CTG

Sabrina Kuah and Geoff Matthews

Introduction

Continuous electronic fetal monitoring (EFM) was developed in the 1960s, and the CTG became commercially available at that time. Erich Saling developed fetal blood sampling prior to CTG, although it subsequently found a place as an adjunct to CTG, and its relevance is now being re-evaluated. Fetal blood sampling has not been shown to reduce caesarean section rates or any prespecified neonatal outcomes.[1]

The CTG has become ubiquitous in modern labour wards, while attempts to validate its role in improving perinatal outcomes have proved challenging.

Fetal ECG has recently become available – the technique involves computerized analysis of the fetal ST waveform and aims, in conjunction with CTG, to provide EFM with more robust specificity and sensitivity.

The human factor has increasingly been recognized as a potential weak link in fetal monitoring and a variety of mitigations proposed. Even when employing standard scoring systems, CTG suffers significantly from intra- and inter-observer variation.[2] Emphasis on systematized training in fetal monitoring for all clinical staff with regular credentialing has become a feature of many delivery suites seeking standardized care. Physiologically based CTG training has been proposed as an alternative approach to reliance on simple pattern recognition.

Computerized decision support technology has been developed with the aim of improving recognition of abnormal fetal heart rate (FHR) patterns and reducing times to effective interventions. Preliminary findings appear encouraging, so clinicians eagerly await the completion of ongoing clinical trials into the effectiveness of this technology.[2]

Cardiotocography

CTG is simply the fetal heart expressed over time, displayed in the patient's room, and in some units, it is also monitored centrally. The heart rate, its variability, the presence or absence of accelerations and decelerations are all assessed by the human observer and the CTG thus interpreted. Traditionally, pattern recognition of the CTG raises suspicions of fetal metabolic acidosis, triggering an attempt to improve the fetal environment, seek reassurance or expedite delivery.

CTG monitoring has become a routine part of clinical obstetric care, although its sensitivity and specificity at detecting fetal metabolic acidosis is poor. The negative predictive value of a normal CTG is in excess of 90 per cent, although the longevity of 'reassurance'

Handbook of CTG Interpretation: From Patterns to Physiology, ed. Edwin Chandraharan. Published by Cambridge University Press. © Cambridge University Press 2017.

obtained is unclear and potentially only for the period the monitoring is ongoing. However, the positive predictive value of an abnormal CTG is quite poor and overall CTG in labour has a false-positive rate of around 60 per cent if acidosis is defined as pH <7.20.

The high false-positive rate of CTG has thus been implicated in the escalating rate of caesarean section births observed in recent decades. While there has been data to suggest a reduction in rates of neonatal seizures, there is, as yet, no level-one evidence of reduction in rates of fetal metabolic acidosis at birth as a result of deployment of CTGs in maternity units.

Adjuncts to CTG

Fetal Blood Sampling

Fetal blood is collected from the scalp and run through a blood gas analyser to obtain a pH and more recently a lactate reading. Management is dictated by the pH result – ≤7.20 has conventionally been used as an indication for delivery.

However, correlating peripheral acidosis detected in fetal scalp blood with central acidosis is flawed since a fetus will progressively protect the central organs (brain, heart and adrenals) at the cost of shutting down the periphery.

Fetal ECG (STAN)

See Chapter 23.

Training and Reducing Human Error

Human error and misinterpretation of CTG data contributes to poor outcomes associated with EFM. Reviews of case series with poor perinatal outcomes have identified significant delay in the recognition of even severe CTG abnormalities.[3] Furthermore, the series suggests that these delays in the recognition of abnormal CTGs are associated with outcomes including cerebral palsy and perinatal death.[4] It would appear that there is an association with clinician seniority. Rates of perinatal mortality in the United Kingdom are significantly increased at times of lesser senior staffing such as at night and in the summer months when many senior staff are on leave.[5]

Credentialing of all staff members in a recognized CTG competency-based training program has increasingly become the norm. The content of training may influence effectiveness, and a physiologically based training rather than pattern recognition has been proposed as preferable.[6]

The Royal Colleges are increasingly standardizing CTG training. In South Australia, all obstetric doctors and midwives must attend and achieve competency in the Royal Australian and New Zealand College of Obstetrics and Gynaecology Fetal Surveillance Education Program.

There is some evidence that intensive CTG training can at least temporarily reduce the proportion of substandard CTG interpretation in cases of low apgars, but the improvement seems to require continued intensive CTG training to be sustained over time.[7]

Computerized Decision Support

Human factors come into play around the issues of uniform recognition of abnormal CTG patterns triggering appropriate decision points. Decision support technology allows for the

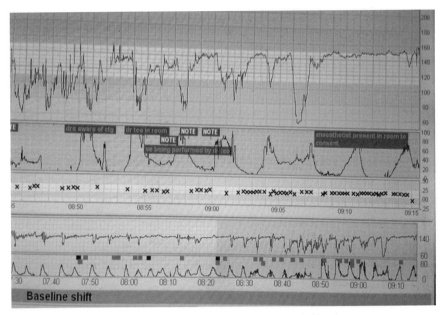

Figure 24.1 Computerized CTG highlighting the onset of a 'baseline shift' to clinicians.

central alerting of an abnormal CTG trace to busy delivery suite staff and suggests a possible interpretation (Figure 24.1). Most systems require attending staff to acknowledge the alert, facilitating a forcing function for clinician's review of the CTG.

While human error can be mitigated by improved training and credentialing, experience from a range of areas including aviation suggests that even the most highly trained operators will potentially benefit from decision support whether it comes from a colleague and/ or computer.

Computerized CTG has been available in various formats since the 1990s and incorporates a decision support capability. Automated analysis of CTG tracings requires processing uterine contraction signals, short-term variability, estimation of FHR baseline, detection of accelerations, abnormal and mean long-term variability and detection and classification of decelerations. Algorithms calculate these variables based on preprogrammed system-specific criteria. Omniview Sis-Porto and the K2 Medical Systems Data Collection System (Guardian)[8] are two currently available commercial systems.

In 2010, a Cochrane Review of antenatal CTG noted that computerized CTG in two studies (469 patients) significantly reduced the relative risk of perinatal mortality (RR 0.2; 95% CI 0.04–0.88).[2] Similarly, intrapartum computerized CTG studies from the 1990s suggest that the software being assessed performed as well as expert obstetricians in interpreting CTGs and predicted poor outcome sooner than the experts.[9]

There are currently two large clinical trials underway assessing two systems of computerized clinical support, the INFANT study (Intelligent Fetal Assessment Monitoring) and the Omniview Sis-Porto trial.

The INFANT trial[10] is randomizing approximately 46,000 patients in units throughout the United Kingdom and is powered to detect a 50 per cent relative risk reduction (5 per cent significance) in a composite score of 'poor perinatal outcome' between those randomized

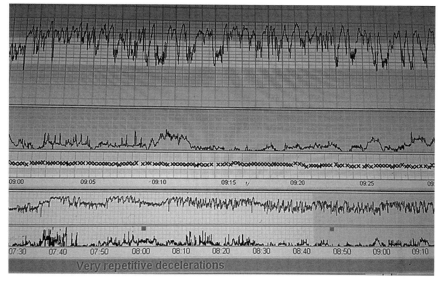

Figure 24.2 The Omniview Sis-Porto decision support software. Note that the computer is flagging up 'very repetitive decelerations' in amber. More severe abnormalities will be highlighted in red.

to decision support and those receiving standard care. This trial is utilizing the 'Guardian' system developed by the Plymouth Group.

The Omniview Sis-Porto system also has decision support software and provides visual and auditory alerts based on the interpretation of CTG but also incorporates fetal ECG (STAN) data (Figure 24.2). The software analyses the CTG–fetal ST and produces a colour-coded alert notifying the operator when there are characteristics that may increase the likelihood of fetal hypoxia. The colour-coded alerts produce management advice (e.g. consider discontinuing/reducing oxytocin infusion or acute tocolysis) depending on the severity of abnormality.

The Omniview Sis-Porto trial has randomized 8,133 women and is powered (5 per cent significance) to detect a 1 per cent reduction in the overall rate of fetal metabolic acidosis from 2.8 per cent to 1.8 per cent. The secondary outcome measures include rate of caesarean section for nonreassuring fetal state; fetal blood sampling rates; operative vaginal delivery rates; apgar scores <7; and admission to neonatal intensive care.

Conclusion

Improved perinatal outcomes may be achieved with intensive physiology-based CTG education for all staff provided there is systematic and sustained effort at credentialing participants.

Fetal ECG ST analysis adds fetal cardiac oxygen metabolism as a second parameter to the existing CTG data, potentially allowing for greater specificity and sensitivity in fetal monitoring.

The incorporation of computerized decision support to the CTG ± fetal ECG mitigates human factors and may provide an opportunity to realize greater dividends from EFM. However, preliminary data from both the Sis-Porto Trial and the Infant Trial which have been presented at scientific meetings (i.e. pending publications) suggest that the use of 'decision-support' computerised systems have not resulted in any significant improvements in perinatal outcomes. This illustrates the importance of using the knowledge of fetal physiology to interpret CTG Traces.

References

1. Alfirevic Z, Devane D, Gyte GML. Continuous cardiotocography (CTG) as a form of electronic fetal monitoring (EFM) for fetal assessment during labour. *Cochrane Database Syst Rev* 2013;5:CD006066.

2. Grivell RM, Alfirevic Z, Gyte GML, Devane D. Antenatal cardiotocography for fetal assessment. *Cochrane Database Syst Rev* 2010;1:CD007863.

3. Ennis M, Vincent CA. Obstetric accidents: a review of 64 cases. *BMJ* 1990;300:1365–7.

4. Gaffney G, Sellers S, Flavell V, Squire M, Johnson A. Case-control study of intrapartum care, cerebral palsy, and perinatal death. *BMJ* 1994;308:743–50.

5. Stewart JH, Andrews J, Cartlidge PH. Numbers of deaths related to intrapartum asphyxia and timing of birth in all Wales Perinatal Survey, 1993–5. *BMJ* 1998;316:657–60.

6. Khangura T, Chandraharan E. Electronic fetal heart rate monitoring: the future. *Curr Women's Health Rev* 2013;9:169–74.

7. Young P, Hamilton R, Hodgett S, Moss M, Rigby C, Jones P, et al. Reducing risk by improving standards of intrapartum fetal care. *J R Soc Med* 2001;94:226–31.

8. Ayres-de-Campos D, Bernardes J, Garrido A, Marques-de-Sá J, Pereira-Leite L. SisPorto 2.0: a program for automated analysis of cardiotocograms. *J Matern Fetal Med* 2000;9:311–18.

9. Keith RDF, Beckley S, Garibaldi JM, Westgate JA, Ifeachor EC, Greene KR. A multicenter comparative study of 17 experts and an intelligent computer system for managing labour using the cardiotocogram. *Br J Obstet Gynaecol* 1995;102:688–700.

10. Brocklehurst P. A multicentre randomized controlled trial of an intelligent system to support decision making in the management of labour using the cardiotocogram (INFANT). Protocol 2014. Version 12. www.ucl.ac.uk/ctu/infant

Peripheral Tests of Fetal Well-being

Charis Mills and Edwin Chandraharan

Key Facts

- Labour is a stressful process for the fetus, and the vast majority of fetuses mount a successful compensatory response to mechanical or hypoxic stresses without sustaining any neurological injury.
- Intrapartum fetal hypoxia leading to fetal decompensation may be associated with adverse perinatal outcomes and long-term neurological sequelae such as cerebral palsy.
- Due to the high false-positive rate of CTG (60–90 per cent), peripheral tests of fetal well-being (fetal scalp blood sampling [FBS], fetal scalp lactate analysis and fetal pulse oximetry) were developed to reduce intrapartum operative interventions.
- Peripheral tests of fetal well-being are not to be used in isolation but are adjuncts to continuous fetal monitoring using CTG.
- This chapter evaluates the current scientific evidence to support the use of these additional tests of fetal well-being in improving neonatal outcomes.

Fetal Scalp Blood Sampling

- FBS was first introduced in 1962 by Erich Saling to estimate fetal acid–base status as an indicator of hypoxia prior to the introduction of CTG into clinical practice.[1] FBS involves the introduction of an amnioscope into the woman's vagina. The fetal scalp is then visualized and a sample of capillary blood is taken via a small puncture wound in the fetal scalp and is analysed for pH (or lactate).
- Unfortunately, the value of estimating capillary blood pH from a peripheral tissue is often inaccurate as the site of fetal scalp sampling is not representative of true acid–base balance. Moreover, the fetal scalp may be compressed during labour and the presence of caput succedaneum may lead to inaccurate results.[2] This may result in unnecessary interventions in fetuses that are not truly hypoxic.
- A Cochrane Systematic Review of 13 studies on fetal heart monitoring found no evidence from the studies that FBS reduces caesarean section rates or neonatal seizures.[3] In addition, there was no evidence of improvement in long-term neurological outcomes.
- However, the Intrapartum Guidelines of the National Institute for Health and Clinical Excellence (NICE) in 2014 still recommends the use of FBS for a pathological CTG, even though the Guideline Development Group has concluded that FBS actually

Handbook of CTG Interpretation: From Patterns to Physiology, ed. Edwin Chandraharan. Published by Cambridge University Press. © Cambridge University Press 2017.

Table 25.1 NICE classification of fetal blood sample results[4]

Scalp pH	Scalp lactate	Interpretation
≥7.25	≤4.1	Normal
>7.21–7.24	4.2–4.8	Borderline
≤7.20	≥4.9	Abnormal

increases the number of caesarean sections and instrumental vaginal deliveries.[4] There is no robust scientific evidence from randomized controlled trials (RCTs) to support reduction in neonatal acidosis.

- FBS does not distinguish between respiratory and metabolic acidaemia. Metabolic acidaemia is associated with neonatal morbidity. FBS is contraindicated in active maternal infection including HIV and herpes and in known or suspected fetal blood disorders.
- Published data in the United Kingdom suggests that it takes 18 minutes to get FBS results, and therefore, in cases of subacute hypoxia, the use of FBS may delay delivery and worsen perinatal outcomes.
- Scientific evidence suggests that the presence of meconium staining of amniotic fluid as well as contamination with normal amniotic fluid itself may result in erroneous values.[5]

Fetal Scalp Lactate Analysis

- Lactate is a metabolite in anaerobic metabolism and reflects tissue hypoxia. Fetal scalp lactate can be obtained via the same method as FBS for pH, but lactate is analysed rather than pH. Table 25.1 shows the NICE classification of fetal blood sample results for both pH and lactate analysis.[4] Repeat sampling and intervention is based on the interpretation of the result, CTG trace, rate of progress of labour and any clinical maternal or fetal indications.
- A large multicentre Swedish RCT including 2,992 women compared lactate analysis versus pH analysis of fetal scalp blood samples to determine the effectiveness for each analysis and management of intrapartum fetal distress and prevention of acidaemia at birth. This study found no significant differences in rates of metabolic acidaemia at birth, Apgar score <7 at 5 minutes of life and rates of operative deliveries for fetal distress between lactate and pH analysis. Failure rates of achieving a sample were higher in the pH group.[6] In other studies, sampling and analysis is found to be more successful and quicker when using fetal lactate analysis. Fetal lactate requires a smaller amount of blood (5 µL) than fetal pH (30–50 µL).
- A recent Cochrane Systematic Review has also confirmed that although fetal scalp lactate was easier to perform and required a smaller scalp blood sample compared to FBS, there was no difference in operative interventions and perinatal outcomes.[7]

Fetal Pulse Oximetry

- Fetal pulse oximetry is an intrapartum test of fetal well-being that involves attachment of a probe to the fetal head to measure oxygen saturation in fetal blood. Fetal pulse oximetry relies on differential rates of absorption of infrared beam of light by oxygenated and deoxygenated haemoglobin at two different wavelengths during an arterial pulsation cycle. Fetal acidaemia is rare when arterial oxygen saturation is >30 per cent; therefore, a SpO_2 >30 per cent is associated with good fetal outcome.

- Technical difficulties include positioning of the probe against fetal cheek and incorrect reading due to the presence of meconium and blood in amniotic fluid.
- A recent Cochrane Review of seven RCTs, involving a total of 8,013 women, showed that fetal pulse oximetry in conjunction with CTG does not improve caesarean section rates compared with the use of CTG alone. One trial comparing oximetry and CTG with CTG and fetal ECG showed an increase in caesarean section rates in the fetal pulse oximetry group.[8]

Recommended Management

- Understand fetal physiology and employ regular CTG review and training to avoid misinterpretation of CTG traces leading to unnecessary intervention in fetuses that are not subject to hypoxia.
- Where possible, if a CTG trace is nonreassuring, seek senior obstetric and midwifery advice and use other additional tests that determine the oxygenation of a central organ such as fetal ECG (STAN) rather than a peripheral test (FBS and pulse oximetry).

Consequences of Mismanagement

- Multiple and failed attempts at FBS for pH and lactate analysis can cause delay in delivery. Recent scientific evidence suggests that it may double the caesarean section rate.[9]
- Failure to understand the pathophysiology of intrapartum fetal hypoxia may result in a delay in delivery due to attempting FBS and thereby worsening perinatal outcomes.
- Rare complications of FBS (fetal scalp pH and lactate) include haemorrhage, sepsis and leakage of cerebrospinal fluid.[10]
- Peripheral tests of fetal well-being can lead to unnecessary maternal and fetal interventions to fetuses that are not subjected to a hypoxic insult. A recent Commentary in 2016 has questioned the ethical and moral issues arising due to some national guidelines continuing to recommend FBS in routine clinical practice without any scientific evidence of benefit but with potential harm.[11]

References

1. Bretscher J, Saling E. pH values in the human fetus during labour. *American Journal of Obstetrics and Gynaecology* 1967;97:906–11.

2. Chandraharan E. Fetal scalp blood sampling during labour: is it a useful diagnostic test or a historical test that no longer has a place in modern clinical obstetrics? *BJOG* 2014. Aug; 121(9):1056–60.

3. Alfirevic Z, Devane D, Gyte GML. Continuous cardiotocography (CTG) as a form of electronic fetal monitoring (EFM) for fetal assessment during labour. *Cochrane Database of Systematic Reviews* 2013;5:CD006066.

4. National Institute for Health and Clinical Excellence (NICE) 2014 Guidelines.

5. Losch A, Kainz C, Kohlberger P, et al. Influence on fetal blood pH when adding amniotic fluid: an in vitro model. *BJOG* 2003;110:453–6.

6. Wiberg-Itzel E, Lipponer C, Normaln M, et al. Determination of pH or lactate in fetal scalp blood in management of

intrapartum fetal distress: randomised controlled multicentre trial. *BMJ* 2008; June 7336(7656):1284–7.

7. East CE, Leader LR, Sheehan P, et al. Intrapartum fetal scalp lactate sampling for fetal assessment in the presence of a non-reassuring fetal heart rate trace. *Cochrane Database Systematic Review* 2010;CD006174.

8. East CE, Begg L, Colditz PB, et al. Fetal pulse oximetry for fetal assessment in labor. *Cochrane Database of Systematic Reviews* 2014;10;CD004075.

9. Holzmann M, Wretler S, Cnattingius S, et al. Neonatal outcomes and delivery mode in labours with repetitive fetal scalp blood sampling. *European Journal of Obstetric Gynaecology Reproductive Biology* 2015;184:97–102.

10. Schaap TP, Moormann KA, Becker JH, et al. Cerebrospinal fluid leakage, an uncommon complication of fetal blood sampling: a case report and review of the literature. *Obstetric Gynecology Survey* 2011;66:42–6.

11. Chandraharan E. Should national guidelines continue to recommend fetal scalp blood sampling during labor? *Journal of Maternal-Fetal & Neonatal Medicine* 2016 Feb 24:1–4.

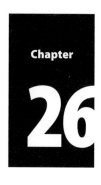

Operative Interventions for Fetal Compromise

Mary Catherine Tolcher and Kyle D. Traynor

Key Facts

- The use of vacuum or forceps can result in apparent deterioration in fetal status (usually prolonged fetal deceleration) when traction is applied.
- Failed operative vaginal delivery is associated with increased neonatal morbidity and necessitates emergent caesarean delivery.

Operative Vaginal Delivery

- Operative vaginal delivery with either vacuum or forceps can serve as a useful alternative to caesarean delivery when a delivery is required during the second stage of labour.
- Common indications for operative intervention include suspected fetal compromise, prolonged second stage of labour, fetal malposition, maternal paraplegia, known contraindication to valsalva (pushing) including cardiovascular or neurological disease, or maternal exhaustion.[1]
- Prerequisites *must be met* prior to attempts at operative vaginal delivery. Clinical criteria outlined in National Institute for Health and Care Excellence (NICE) guidelines include vertex presentation, full dilation, ruptured membranes, clinically adequate pelvis and knowledge of fetal position. Other important elements include informed consent, adequate skills on the part of the operator and availability of staff and facilities for caesarean delivery if required.[2]
- Additionally, the preparation for complications including shoulder dystocia and postpartum haemorrhage should be undertaken. Personnel trained in neonatal resuscitation should be present for delivery.

Anticipated CTG Changes Following Instrument Application

- Following the application of a vacuum with suction to pressures up to 600 mm Hg,[3] fetal heart rate (FHR) decelerations can be expected. This phenomenon is explained by known mechanisms of FHR regulation including the interaction of the sympathetic and parasympathetic nervous systems. When suction is applied to the fetal head, the increased intracranial pressure results in increased systemic vascular resistance which stimulates baroreceptors in the fetal heart to activate the vagus nerve and slow the

Handbook of CTG Interpretation: From Patterns to Physiology, ed. Edwin Chandraharan. Published by Cambridge University Press. © Cambridge University Press 2017.

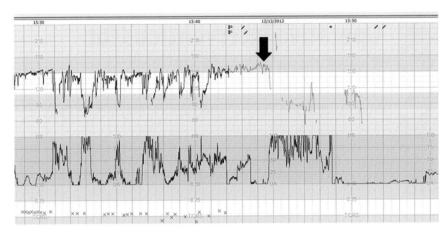

Figure 26.1 Acute drop in FHR following the removal of fetal scalp electrode and application of the vacuum cup (arrow). This precipitous fall in FHR is *not* secondary to hypoxia but due to an intense parasympathetic stimulation.

FHR.[4,5] In addition, there may be direct stimulation of parasympathetic nerve endings on the fetal scalp resulting in a prolonged deceleration.

- Anticipated effects following forceps application are similar to those seen with vacuum-assisted delivery as the mechanism of increased intracranial pressure is similar (Figure 26.1). Kelly evaluated 62 operative vaginal deliveries including 44 forceps and 18 vacuum deliveries by measuring the intensity of traction in pounds and the effects on FHR during application, traction and posttraction.[6] Fetal decelerations were commonly elicited when traction was applied to either instrument (84 per cent).
- Scientific evidence suggests that the reflex cardiac deceleration is triggered when intracranial pressure exceeds 40 mm Hg.

Failed Operative Vaginal Delivery

- While the goal of vacuum or forceps is to achieve a vaginal delivery, not all attempts are successful. Attempted vacuum-assisted vaginal delivery is more likely to result in a failed trial of operative vaginal delivery as compared to forceps (7.5 per cent versus 1.4 per cent in one study and 15.7 per cent versus 0.4 per cent in another).[7,8]
- Risk factors for failed trial include maternal body mass index over 30 kg/m^2, estimated fetal weight >4,000 g, occipito-posterior position and midcavity delivery or when more than one-fifth of the fetal head is palpable per abdomen.[2] Other potential contributors to a failed attempt include fetal caput succedaneum, hair, asynclitism/malposition and improper instrument placement.[3]
- According to current guidelines, operative vaginal delivery should be abandoned when there is no evidence of progressive descent with the application of moderate traction during each uterine contraction. Alternatively, further attempts at operative vaginal delivery should be abandoned if delivery is not imminent following three contractions in which traction was applied using a correctly placed instrument by an experienced operator.[2] No more than three vacuum pop-offs has also been suggested.[3]

- When attempts at operative vaginal delivery have failed, the subsequent caesarean delivery can be complicated by a deeply impacted fetal head. Forces exerted to deliver the fetus may compound effects on increased intracranial pressures. Further, uterine contractions or fetal malposition can make delivery difficult.
- Uterine relaxants and disengagement techniques including the push (vaginal hand from below) and pull (reverse breech extraction) methods have been described.[9] Care must be taken to prevent hysterotomy extensions resulting in excessive blood loss and fetal injury. Reported fetal injuries associated with difficult fetal extraction at the time of caesarean include long bone and skull fractures.[9]
- Delivery by caesarean may be essential if the likelihood of a failed operative vaginal delivery is deemed high based on clinical circumstances and experience of the operator.

Decision to Delivery Interval

Risks of intracranial haemorrhage, facial nerve injury, convulsions, central nervous system depression and mechanical ventilation are significantly higher in infants delivered by caesarean delivery following a failed attempt at operative vaginal delivery than in those delivered spontaneously.[10]

- Because of known increased neonatal morbidity associated with failed trial of operative vaginal delivery, expeditious delivery by caesarean is essential, especially if there are features suggestive of fetal decompensation on the CTG. According to NICE guidelines, caesarean delivery following a failed trial of operative vaginal delivery is considered category 1 (emergent) and should occur as soon as possible, generally within 30 minutes as an audit standard.[2]
- According to one study of operative vaginal deliveries in Scotland, of 998 operative vaginal deliveries attempted, 965 were successful (96.7 per cent).[8] Of the 965 successful operative vaginal deliveries, 798 were performed in the labour room (82.7 per cent) with a decision to delivery interval of 14.5 minutes (SD 9.5), while 167 were performed in the operating room (17.3 per cent) with a decision to delivery interval of 30.3 minutes (SD 14.1).

Pitfalls

- Misapplication of instrument due to incorrect diagnosis of fetal position.
- Choice of wrong instrument (use of a nonrotational forceps for a malrotated fetal head).
- Prolonged attempts at failed trial of operative vaginal delivery (e.g. greater than three pop-offs with vacuum or use of multiple instruments).
- Abandonment of trial of operative vaginal delivery due to fetal decelerations with traction.
- Failure to effect delivery by caesarean expeditiously in cases of failed trial of operative vaginal delivery if there are features suggestive of fetal decompensation on the CTG trace.
- Inadequate management of an impacted fetal head at the time of caesarean delivery following a failed trial of operative vaginal delivery leading to fetal trauma and increased intracranial pressure resulting in a reduction in carotid circulation.

Consequences of Mismanagement

- Failed instrumental delivery due to the use of excessive/inappropriate force after observing a deceleration secondary to expected parasympathetic stimulation after the application of forceps or vacuum cup.
- Fetal complications may occur secondary to an unnecessary operative vaginal delivery due to overreaction to patterns observed on the CTG trace without understanding the fetal physiological response to on-going hypoxic or mechanical stress. These complications include cephalohematoma, fetal intracranial haemorrhage, fetal skull fracture and delayed caesarean delivery.
- Angle extensions and excessive blood loss during caesarean delivery secondary to misinterpretation of the CTG trace during advanced second stage of labour.
- Fetal neurological injury or perinatal death due to a delay in accomplishing delivery despite ongoing features on the CTG trace suggestive of decompensation of the brain (loss of baseline FHR variability) or the myocardium (unstable baseline FHR or a prolonged deceleration with loss of baseline variability within deceleration).

References

1. Unzila AA, Norwitz ER. Vacuum-assisted vaginal delivery. *Rev Obstet Gynecol* 2009;2(1):5–17.

2. Royal College of Obstetricians and Gynaecologists. *Green-top guideline 26: Operative vaginal delivery*. London: RCOG; 2011.

3. Kiwi Complete Vacuum Delivery System with Palm Pump. Clinical Innovations. *Instructions for use*. www.clinicalinnovations.com/site_files/files/Kiwi%20IFU.pdf. Accessed 26 March 2015.

4. Nageotte MP. Intrapartum fetal surveillance. Chapter In: *Creasy and Resnik's maternal-fetal medicine: principles and practice*, 33, 488-506.e2. Elsevier 2014.

5. Zilianti M, Cabello F, Estrada MA. Fetal heart rate patterns during forceps operation. *J Perinat Med* 1978;6:80–86.

6. Kelly JV. Instrumental delivery and the fetal heart rate. *Am J Obstet Gynecol* 1963;87:529–37.

7. Al-Kadri H, Sabr Y, Al-Saif S, Abulaimoun B, Ba'Aqeel H, Saleh A. Failed individual and sequential instrumental vaginal delivery: contributing risk factors and maternal-neonatal complications. *Acta Obstet Gynecol Scand* 2003;82(7):642–8.

8. Murphy DJ, Koh DKM. Cohort study of the decision to delivery interval and neonatal outcome for emergency operative vaginal delivery. *Am J Obstet Gynecol* 2007;196:145.e1-145.e7.

9. Berhan Y, Berhan A. A meta-analysis of reverse breech extraction to deliver a deeply impacted head during cesarean delivery. *Int J Gynaecol Obstet* 2014;124(2):99–105.

10. Towner D, Castro MA, Eby-Wilkens E, Gilbert WM. Effect of mode of delivery in nulliparous women on neonatal intracranial injury. *N Engl J Med* 1999;341(23):1709–14.

Nonhypoxic Causes of CTG Changes

Dovilé Kalvinskaité and Edwin Chandraharan

The fetal heart rate (FHR) is controlled through various integrated physiological mechanisms, most importantly through an interaction of sympathetic and parasympathetic nervous systems. Optimum functioning of the fetal heart requires an intact central nervous system and a well-developed fetal heart to respond adequately. Thus, abnormal CTG changes may be caused by congenital malformations or organic changes in the fetal brain or heart, together with infection and other metabolic changes that might affect these organs (Figures 27.1 and 27.2).

Key Facts

- Various congenital, organic or metabolic changes in the fetus may cause an abnormal FHR pattern, in the absence of hypoxia.
- Up to 75 per cent of fetuses with nonhypoxic CNS damage represent changes in CTG, even though there is no single unique feature on the CTG trace associated with such an abnormality.
- 'Nonreassuring' FHR patterns are more common in preterm fetuses because their brain is less well developed. Such CTG abnormalities may occur in up to 60 per cent of these cases.
- Maternal administration with various medications may affect the fetus and modulate the CTG changes.
- Erroneous monitoring of MHR as FHR may also result in CTG changes (see Chapter 6).

Key Features on the CTG Trace

- Fetuses with normal neurological state have quiet sleep and active periods termed 'cycling'. Absence of cycling may be due to major fetal brain malformation or haemorrhage, fetal infection or medication.
- Reduced or absent baseline variability is the most common feature seen in the CTG when the CNS function is impaired due to congenital malformation or fetal infection. It can also be caused by medications and occurs shortly after administering them.
- A persistently 'flat' baseline variability with normal baseline FHR and without accelerations or decelerations may reflect a severe pre-existing neurological damage (Figure 27.3). The fetus, therefore, is unlikely to be hypoxic if a decreased variability

Handbook of CTG Interpretation: From Patterns to Physiology, ed. Edwin Chandraharan. Published by Cambridge University Press. © Cambridge University Press 2017.

Nonhypoxic Brain Damage

Preterm fetus

- Periventricular Leucomalacia (white matter injury) - white matter around the ventricles is highly metabolically active and may be injured due to inflammatory mediators or haemorrhage

Preterm and term fetus

- Congenital malformations of the fetal brain
- Cerebral vascular accidents (e.g. intra-uterine fetal stroke)
- Selective neuronal necrosis (usually secondary to the occlusion of a blood vessel)
- Fetal trauma (intracranial haemorrhage secondary to forceps)
- Inflammatory damage (maternal infection, chorioamnionitis, fetal sepsis, meningitis, encephalitis)
- Fetal metabolic disorders
- Maternal metabolic disorders (e.g. diabetes ketoacidosis)
- Medications (e.g. analgesics, opioids, tranquilizers, magnesium sulpahte, barbiturates, methyldopa)

Figure 27.1 Causes of nonhypoxic brain injuries.

Nonhypoxic Myocardial Damage with CTG Changes

Electrical

- Tachyarrythmias (sinus tachycardia, SVT, atrial flutter)
- Bradyarrhythmias (second degree and complete AV block, long QT syndrome)

Nonelectrical

- Immunological (maternal SLE, rheumatoid arthritis, dermatomyositis, Sjögren's syndrome)
- Medications (affecting mycordial function or conduction)
- Structural malformations of the heart

Figure 27.2 Causes of nonhypoxic myocardial damage.

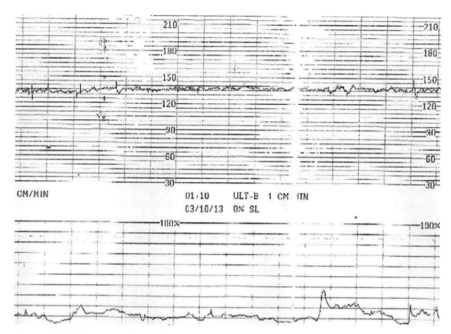

Figure 27.3 CTG trace of a fetus with a massive intracranial haemorrhage in the antenatal period. Note the total absence of baseline variability and absence of preexisting decelerations.

develops in the absence of preceding decelerations. The lack of baseline variability may also correlate with the severity of fetal brain damage.

- An increase in baseline FHR can be due to maternal infection, chorioamnionitis or fetal infection. Other major causes of fetal tachycardia are cardiac arrhythmias and maternal administration of sympathetic (e.g. terbutaline) or parasympathetic (e.g. atropine) medications and maternal hyperthyroidism.
- The most common fetal tachyarrhythmia is supraventricular tachycardia (SVT), which is characterized by a persistent tachycardia at FHR of 210 to 320 bpm with reduced baseline variability. SVT usually appears around 28 to 30 weeks of gestation, and if it is persistent at a rate of >230 bpm, it can lead to the development of hydrops fetalis.
- Baseline FHR bradycardia can be caused by maternal administration of drugs (labetolol, atenolol), prolonged maternal hypoglycaemia or hypothermia, connective tissue diseases, fetal cardiac conduction or anatomic defects. As long as normal baseline variability is present, fetal bradycardia may be considered benign in such cases. Intermittent fetal bradycardia frequently is due to congenital heart block. Even in cases of complete heart block, the FHR does not go below 55–60 bpm (ventricular rate); if it does, a coexisting fetal hypoxia should be excluded. The baseline variability will be lost within deceleration in cases of hypoxia due to a reduction in cerebral circulation.
- Pseudo-sinusoidal fetal heart pattern may be observed following the administration of meperidine, morphine, and it should resolve within 30 minutes. A true sinusoidal trace may occur with fetal intracranial haemorrhage, chorioamnionitis or severe maternal diabetes.
- Unsteady baseline rate or 'wandering' baseline can be due to a severe brain or cardiac malformation and may appear as a preterminal event.

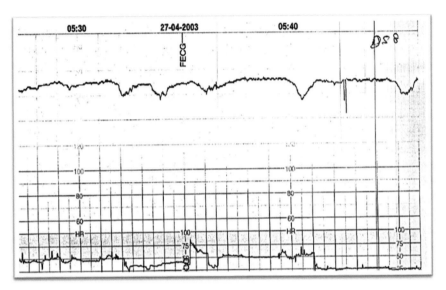

Figure 27.4 Total loss of baseline variability due to a severe fetal CNS infection.

Key Pathophysiology behind Patterns Seen on the CTG Trace

- Decreased or absent variability occurs when the autonomic nervous system, which is responsible for the modularity function of the CNS, is impaired. Hence, severe malformations or organic changes (e.g. large cerebral haemorrhage) in the midbrain or cortex (Figure 27.1) – or when central neural pathways are disorganized because of chromosomal or other genetic abnormalities – abnormal features may be observed on the CTG trace.

- Increase in sympathetic or decrease in parasympathetic nervous system tone causes fetal tachycardia. It can be due to a direct fetal infection or as a secondary fetal response due to transplacental passage of pyrogens in the presence of maternal infection, as well as due to fetal cardiac electrical abnormalities, medications or maternal anxiety (release of adrenaline).

- Fetus exposure to an infection may cause a fetal inflammatory response syndrome which leads to the development of cytokine-mediated white matter injury in the fetal brain and, therefore, changes in the CTG (Figure 27.4).

- Fetal heart conduction defects usually are associated with maternal connective tissue diseases, because maternal SS-A/Ro and SS-B/La antibodies cause inflammatory myocarditis and disrupts fetal cardiac conduction system.

- If there is a derangement or a virtual absence of CNS control over the FHR, a sinusoidal pattern is observed.

- Intrauterine convulsions may result in repeated accelerations with the absence of cycling (Figure 27.5). Repeated 'low-amplitude' accelerations secondary to disorganized fetal movements during convulsions with absence of cycling should alert clinicians to ongoing intrauterine convulsions (Figure 27.5). In this case, the umbilical cord gases would be entirely normal, but the neonate may continue to have neonatal convulsions. An MRI scan may not show any evidence of hypoxic injury.

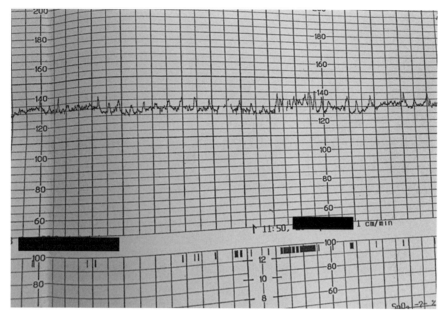

Figure 27.5 CTG trace in intrauterine fetal convulsions. Note the absence of cycling and repeated 'low-amplitude' accelerations secondary to disorganized fetal movements during convulsions.

Recommended Management

- Hypoxic causes and maternal or fetal infection that may have resulted in nonreassuring CTG changes must be excluded.
- If the fetus is unlikely to be hypoxic and there are no other causes to explain nonreassuring features observed on the CTG trace, a further detailed investigation should be performed (e.g. ultrasound to confirm congenital malformations, fetal echocardiography).
- SVT and fetal heart block require an active management and may be associated with fetal compromise and/or maternal disease. Most other cardiac arrhythmias, although, are considered as benign and do not require immediate delivery or other than management targeted at a specific condition (e.g. sympatholytic drugs to correct supraventricular tachycardia).
- In cases of complete fetal heart block, a search for autoimmune antibodies in mother's blood should be performed even if she is asymptomatic.
- FHR changes which develop after administration of drugs can be managed expectantly.

Key tips to Optimize the Outcome

- The whole clinical picture and previous CTG traces have to be considered to exclude ongoing nonhypoxic causes of fetal injury.
- One has to make sure that the CTG trace is normal with no evidence of hypoxia before giving any medications.

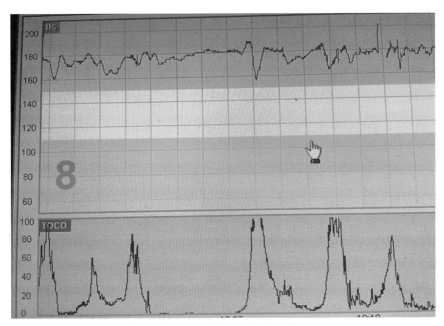

Figure 27.6 CTG trace in a fetus with severe cardiac conduction defects.

- If a nonhypoxic cause (e.g. intrauterine infection, intrauterine convulsions or cardiac rhythm abnormality) is suspected, the neonatal team should be informed in advance to optimize outcome after birth.
- Women should be counselled regarding the prognosis of the suspected/diagnosed nonhypoxic cause of fetal injury as well as the role and limitations of electronic FHR monitoring.

Pitfalls

- Failure to recognize the absence of cycling on the CTG trace. In the absence of ongoing hypoxia, decelerations may be absent.
- The changes observed on the CTG trace may be misdiagnosed as due to hypoxia leading to unnecessary interventions such as fetal scalp blood sampling or unnecessary emergency caesarean section.
- In the presence of abnormal CTG trace with a confirmed fetal anomaly (Figure 27.4), a true ongoing fetal hypoxia and acidaemia may not be recognized, which may worsen neurological damage to the fetus.
- The use of fetal ECG (STAN) in the presence of cardiac conduction defects (Figure 27.6) as these may influence the waveforms observed on the fetal ECG leading to unnecessary operative interventions.

Consequences of Mismanagement

- Antepartum fetal death.

- Fetal neurological impairment or higher neonatal morbidity rate due to a failure to recognize an ongoing infection.
- A necessary management of a neonate is delayed and neonatal morbidity increased when an underlying fetal brain or cardiac abnormality is not recognized timely before the delivery.
- Early neonatal death.

References

1. Kodoma Y, Sameshima H, Ikeda T, Ikenoue T. Intrapartum fetal heart rate patterns in infants (>34 weeks) with poor neurological outcome. *Early Human Development* 2009;85:235–8.

2. ACOG. Practice Bulletin on Intrapartum fetal heart rate monitoring: nomenclature, interpretation, and general management principles. *American College of Obstetricians and Gynecologists* 2009;106:192–202.

3. Yanamandra N, Chandraharan E. Saltatory and sinusoidal heart rate (FHR) patterns and significance of FHR 'overshoots'. *Current Women's Health Reviews* 2013;9:175–82.

4. McDonnell S, Chandraharan E. Fetal heart rate interpretation in the second stage of labour: pearls and pitfalls. *British Journal of Medicine and Medical Research* 2015;7(12):956–70.

5. Govaert P. Prenatal stroke. *Seminars in Fetal and Neonatal Medicine* 2009;14:250–66.

6. Rovira N, Alarcon A, Iriondo M, Ibanez M, Poo P, Cusi V, Agut T, Pertierra A, Krauel X. Impact of histological chorioamnionitis, funisitis and clinical chorioamnionitis on neurodevelopmental outcome of preterm infants. *Early Human Development* 2010;87:253–7.

7. Kuypers E, Ophelders D, Jellema RK, Kunzmann S, Gavilanes AW, Kramer BW. White matter injury following fetal inflammatory response syndrome induced by chorioamnionitis and fetal sepsis: Lessons from experimental ovine models. *Early Human Development* 2012;88:931–6.

8. Wang X, Rousset CI, Hagberg H, Mallard C. Lipopolysaccharide-induced inflammation and perinatal brain injury. *Science Direct* 2006:11:343–53.

9. Cardiotocograph interpretation: more difficult problems. Chapter in: *Fetal Monitoring in Practice.* 3rd ed. Gibb D, Arulkumaran S. (eds). Elsevier: Churchill Livingstone, 2008.

10. Strasburger JF, Cheulkar B, Wichman HJ. Perinatal arrhythmias: diagnosis and management. *Clinical Perinatology* 2007;34(4):627–56.

Chapter

28

Neonatal Implications of Intrapartum Fetal Hypoxia

Justin Richards

Introduction

Intermittent fetal hypoxia is an integral part of normal childbirth, and the healthy fetus is extremely well adapted to withstand this unharmed. As the uterine muscle contracts during the process of labour, the blood supply to the placenta is reduced, and oxygen and nutrient delivery to the fetus is reduced. Between uterine contractions, the uterine muscle relaxes and oxygen and nutrient supply is restored. Studies in animals have shown that intermittent, regular and complete interruption of fetal blood supply is well tolerated if these interruptions are shorter in duration and the fetus is given adequate time to recover. This is borne out by what we observe in clinical practice.

When Does Fetal Hypoxia Pose a Risk for the Fetus?

- Despite very effective fetal adaptations to cope with acute oxygen and nutrient deprivation during labour, neonatal brain injury resulting from inadequate oxygen in the perinatal period (perinatal hypoxic-ischaemic encephalopathy [HIE]) is estimated to account for 23 per cent of neonatal deaths worldwide[1] and 9–10 per cent of neonatal deaths in the United Kingdom.[2]
- In babies that survive, a significant number will develop long-term neurological sequelae ranging from mild behavioural disorders to significant cognitive impairment and/or cerebral palsy.
- Fetal asphyxia occurs when inadequate oxygen supply leads to anaerobic respiration and subsequent metabolic acidosis and hyperlactaemia. A mild degree of asphyxia occurs in all normal deliveries with no adverse sequelae; however, the chances of significant injury increase as metabolic acidosis becomes more profound.
- Studies demonstrate that an umbilical cord blood pH <7.0 is associated with an increased risk of brain injury, although even at these levels the majority of babies will recover without long-term effects.
- There are other factors which may reduce the ability of the fetus to cope with hypoxia during delivery. Placental dysfunction is known to be associated with an increased risk of HIE, and chorioamnionitis is more common in the placental histology of babies with HIE, suggesting that inflammation may also be a contributory factor. In babies that develop HIE, having clinical signs of sepsis increases the risk of brain injury.[3,4]

Handbook of CTG Interpretation: From Patterns to Physiology, ed. Edwin Chandraharan. Published by Cambridge University Press. © Cambridge University Press 2017.

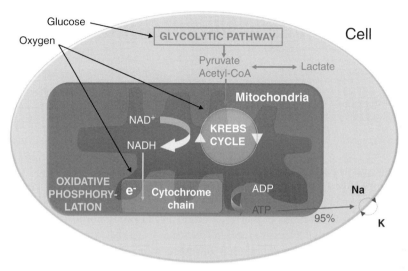

Figure 28.1 Normal cellular energy metabolism demonstrating pathways of ATP production from glucose and oxygen.

- Asphyxia that is severe enough to lead to significant neonatal encephalopathy usually also leads to damage to multiple organ systems in the fetus and newborn. Renal and hepatic impairment are common, but usually recover with time.
- Cardiac dysfunction may lead to hypotension requiring inotropic support and respiratory involvement to pulmonary hypertension and respiratory failure.

Mechanisms of Hypoxic Brain Injury

In normal cellular energy metabolism in the fetal and neonatal brain, glucose is transported into the cell and, through gluconeogenesis and the Krebs cycle, leads to a reduction of NAD to NADH. NADH is used to transport electrons into the respiratory chain which in turn drive oxidative phosphorylation through the reduction of oxygen. The end products are high-energy phosphate compounds (mainly ATP) used to power the cell (Figure 28.1). As part of this process, small quantities of oxygen-free radicals are formed, but in normally functioning cells, these are scavenged through antioxidant mechanisms.

The mechanisms of brain injury following hypoxic insult are complex and involve two stages.

1. Interruption of oxygen and nutrient supply to the fetal brain leads to primary energy failure within minutes. There is a rapid depletion of intracellular ATP stores and ultimately cellular necrosis is caused by a failure of sodium potassium pump if oxygen supply is not restored.
2. Reperfusion following resuscitation leads to a rapid restoration of oxidative phosphorylation. Initially ATP levels return almost to normal; however, a period of secondary energy failure follows, when cellular energy supplies fall again. This is caused by a cascade of cytotoxic reactions within the cell triggered by the processes of reoxygenation.
3. During primary energy failure, electrons accumulate in the mitochondria. When oxygen levels are restored, these electrons combine with oxygen to produce highly reactive

Table 28.1 Clinical grading system for HIE[9]

Grade 1	Grade 2	Grade 3
Irritability hyperalert	Lethargic	Comatose
Mild hypotonia	Marked abnormalities of tone	Severe hypotonia
No seizures	Seizures	Prolonged seizures
Poor sucking	Requires tube feeding	Failure to maintain spontaneous respiration

free radicals that overwhelm the normal cellular antioxidant mechanisms and lead to the production of highly toxic reactive oxygen compounds that damage the intracellular structures.

4. Ultimately these cytotoxic reactions trigger programmed cell death (apoptosis). Current evidence suggests that excessive oxygen levels may exacerbate this process – this is the reason that air is now recommended for resuscitation of the newborn in the first instance.

Clinical Features of Hypoxic-Ischaemic Encephalopathy

- Clinical assessment of a baby following HIE is essential to guide treatment and determine prognosis. In 1976, Sarnat and Sarnat published a staging system for assessment of HIE that classified babies according to examination as stage 1 (mild), 2 (moderate) or 3 (severe).[5] This allowed clinicians to predict the likely outcome of babies with HIE, and a modified version forms the basis of standard assessment to this day (Table 28.1).
- After a severe hypoxic insult, brain activity is initially suppressed during primary energy failure, and clinically the baby is profoundly hypotonic. Reduced brain activity and hypotonia persist through a latent phase often lasting several hours, until the process of secondary energy failure begins.
- During this time, monitoring of brain activity using a cerebral function monitor (CFM) shows reduced cortical activity. Following the latent phase, there is a release of excitatory neurotransmitters within the brain associated with the baby developing seizure activity. In severe HIE and neonatal encephalopathy, seizures often persist for up to 5–7 days, reaching a maximal peak at 1–2 days.[6]

Management of HIE

- The mainstay of treatment for HIE is supportive, with respiratory support, seizure control and implementation of nasogastric tube feeds often required, as well as managing disruption to other organ systems.
- Following the results of recent studies of therapeutic hypothermia,[7] this is now a standard of care for babies with moderate or severe HIE (Sarnat stages 2 or 3) in healthcare environments that are able to provide safe intensive care.[8]
- The CFM may be used to help make a more objective, early assessment of encephalopathy when deciding which babies are likely to benefit from therapeutic hypothermia. Hypothermia is moderate, with the aim to reduce core temperature to between 33°C and 34°C for 72 hours, followed by gradual rewarming.

Table 28.2 Comparison of outcomes for moderate vs severe HIE in the Cochrane meta-analysis of cooling for HIE[7]

Severity of HIE	Outcome	Treatment group	
		Therapeutic hypothermia	Standard care (normothermia)
Moderate(Sarnat stage 2)	Death	33/244 (13%)	53/232 (23%)
	Death or major disability	89/243 (37%)	123/229 (54%)
	Major disability in survivors assessed	56/211 (27%)	70/179 (39%)
Severe(Sarnat stage 3)	Death	75/143 (52%)	96/142 (68%)
	Death or major disability	100/143 (70%)	120/140 (86%)
	Major disability in survivors assessed	26/68 (37%)*	24/47 (51%)*

*These results were not statistically significant in the subgroup analysis.

- MRI scanning 3–7 days after the hypoxic event and EEG/CFM add valuable information to clinical assessment when determining prognosis and are routinely performed in most centres offering therapeutic hypothermia.
- Regular discussions of the condition of the baby and likely outcome with parents are essential throughout the stay in intensive care. In severely affected infants with stage 3 HIE that remain comatose, it is usually appropriate to discuss palliative care with the parents, particularly if CFM/EEG and/or MRI scan show evidence of severe injury with poor prognosis.

Outcomes

- Outcomes for babies with stage 1 HIE are good, with death or disability rates <1 per cent.
- In both moderate and severe encephalopathy (Sarnat stages 2 and 3), rates of death or disability in a recent Cochrane meta-analysis[7] were lower in babies receiving therapeutic hypothermia (Table 28.2).
- Disability includes cerebral palsy and developmental delay as well as hearing and visual disturbances. Overall risk of death or disability in severe HIE remains high despite modern intensive care and therapeutic hypothermia, with only 30 per cent of babies surviving without major disability.[7]

References

1. Newborn death and illness. WHO. Available from: www.who.int/pmnch/media/press_materials/fs/fs_newborndealth_illness/en/

2. Perinatal mortality 2009. CMACE. Available from: http://hqip.org.uk/assets/NCAPOP-Library/CMACE-Reports/35.-March-2011-Perinatal-Mortality-2009.pdf

3. Jenster M, Bonifacio SL, Ruel T, Rogers EE, Tam EW, Partridge JC, et al. Maternal or neonatal infection: association with neonatal encephalopathy outcomes. *Pediatr Res* 2014;76(1):93–9.

4. Wu YW, Colford JM. Chorioamnionitis as a risk factor for cerebral palsy: a meta-analysis. *JAMA* 2000;284(11):1417–24.

5. Sarnat HB, Sarnat MS. Neonatal encephalopathy following fetal distress. A clinical and electroencephalographic study. *Arch Neurol* 1976;33(10):696–705.

6. Wyatt J. Applied physiology: brain metabolism following perinatal asphyxia. *Curr Paediatr* 2002;12(3):227–31.

7. Jacobs SE, Berg M, Hunt R, Tarnow-Mordi WO, Inder TE, Davis PG. Cooling for newborns with hypoxic ischaemic encephalopathy. *Cochrane Database Syst Rev* 2013;1:CD003311.

8. IPG347. Therapeutic hypothermia with intracorporeal temperature monitoring for hypoxic perinatal brain injury. NICE. 2010. Available from: www.nice.org.uk/guidance/ipg347

9. Levene ML, Kornberg J, Williams TH. The incidence and severity of post-asphyxial encephalopathy in full-term infants. *Early Hum Dev* 1985;11(1):21–6.

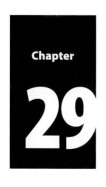

Chapter

29

Role of the Anaesthetist in the Management of Fetal Compromise during Labour

Anuji Amarasekara and Anthony Addei

Fetal asphyxia leads to fetal compromise, which, if not corrected or circumvented, will result in decompensation of physiologic responses (primarily redistribution of blood flow to preserve oxygenation of vital organs) and cause permanent central nervous system damage and other damage or death.

Key Facts

- Anaesthetists participate directly and indirectly in the management of fetal compromise during labour.
- Fetal well-being can be assessed during high-risk labour by electronic FHR monitoring using a CTG to monitor changes in FHR.
- Decelerations and fetal bradycardia have been described after all types of effective labour analgesia (epidural, spinal and combined spinal epidural, and intravenous opioids).
- More dramatic hypoxia-inducing events include placental abruption, cord prolapse and antepartum or intrapartum (fetal) haemorrhage.
- All these may lead to fetal compromise and may necessitate emergency delivery.
- Regardless of the aetiology of FHR abnormalities, it is important to manage these changes correctly when they occur.
- Obstetric cases account for 0.8 per cent of general anaesthetics in the Fifth National Audit Project (NAP5) on Accidental Awareness during General Anaesthesia (AAGA) Activity Survey. However, obstetric cases account for approximately 10 per cent of reports of AAGA, making it the most markedly overrepresented of all surgical specialties.

Key Pathophysiology

- Reduction in oxygen delivery to the fetus is associated with fetal compromise.
  - Metabolic acidosis results from persistent hypoxia via anaerobic metabolism and production of lactic acid.
- Oxygen delivery to the fetus is dependent on maternal circulation, placental transfer and fetal circulation.

Handbook of CTG Interpretation: From Patterns to Physiology, ed. Edwin Chandraharan. Published by Cambridge University Press. © Cambridge University Press 2017.

- Uterine oxygen delivery = uterine blood flow × arterial oxygen content. Uterine blood flow is determined by perfusion pressure (arterial – venous pressure) and resistance.
- Aortocaval compression occurs when the pregnant uterus compresses the inferior vena cava and descending aorta within the abdomen. This can result in reduced blood flow to the utero-placental unit and maternal hypotension. The effect is maximal in supine position.
- In labour, intrauterine pressure increases during contractions. Initially the uterine veins become compressed, and intervillous blood volume increases until intrauterine pressure is sufficient to stop arterial flow.
- Placental oxygen transport occurs along a gradient from maternal to fetal blood.
- Fetal haemoglobin (HbF) has a higher affinity for oxygen than adult haemoglobin. The fetus also has higher haemoglobin, 16.5 g/dL (range, 15–18.6 g/dL), which helps to ensure adequate oxygen content.
- Oxygen carriage to vital organs of the fetus is also dependent on fetal cardiac output and adequate umbilical circulation. Fetal stroke volume is relatively fixed, and FHR is the major determinant of cardiac output.
- Occlusion of the umbilical cord will restrict delivery of oxygenated blood to the fetus via the umbilical vein.

The method of anaesthesia may affect neonatal outcome by transplacental drug transfer and by influencing maternal haemodynamics and hence placental perfusion.

Intrauterine fetal resuscitation (IUFR) can result in significant improvements in the condition of the fetus.

Recommended Management

- Rapid, coordinated, multidisciplinary approach is vital to minimizing fetal compromise that can lead to permanent damage to the baby.
- The anaesthetist has a role in assessing the mother quickly and initiating or continuing resuscitation as required.
- The goal of IUFR is to optimize the fetal condition in utero so that labour may continue safely or to improve fetal well-being prior to emergency delivery.
- IUFR consists of simple (SPOILT) steps:
  - Syntocinon: Stop syntocinon infusion to reduce the intensity and frequency of uterine contractions, leading to improved placental perfusion.
  - Position: Left lateral position of the mother to relieve aortocaval compression and improve venous return and placental perfusion.
  - Oxygen: High-flow oxygen with Hudson mask and reservoir bag to increase maternal oxygen saturation (e.g. in cases of maternal collapse and maternal hypoxia).
  - IV fluids: Rapid fluid infusion to restore maternal vascular volume. This may also help to dilute oxytocin in blood in cases of uterine hyperstimulation.
  - Low BP: Vasopressor (phenylephrine 50 µg – 100 µg increments; or ephedrine 3 mg – 6 mg increments) if low maternal blood pressure.
  - Tocolytics should be used to provide uterine relaxation to improve placental oxygenation if there is evidence of uterine hyperstimulation.

Key Issues

- In cases of significant fetal compromise unresponsive to IUFR, or which show only a transient response, early delivery of the fetus may be indicated. Delivery by a 'category 1' caesarean section may be required.
- The decision as to the method of anaesthesia is a balance between degree of urgency and level of concern about maternal risks of general anaesthesia. In cases of imminent fetal demise, delays may become clinically significant.
- A controversial case series describing 'rapid sequence spinal anaesthesia' as an alternative to general anaesthesia for urgent caesarean section has been published.
- Good communication helps to identify and prepare a plan for at-risk patients on the labour ward who may become an emergency. This may make the difference between the possibility of planned, timely regional anaesthesia and emergency general anaesthetic.
- Obstetric anaesthesia is regarded as a high-risk subspecialty for AAGA.
- Undue haste in situations that are not true emergencies may cause maternal and/or fetal harm due to anaesthesia and surgical complications.

Key Tips to Optimize Outcome

- The use of IUFR is based on an understanding of maternal physiology, oxygen transfer, effects of uterine contractions and evidence from numerous publications in literature.
- Variable decelerations may result from cord compression. Relief of such compression may be achieved by trying several right or left lateral positions.
- Avoid prolonged maternal oxygen administration, which should only be administered in cases of maternal hypoxia and maternal collapse.
- Care must be taken to avoid fluid overload in fluid-restricted patients (e.g. preeclampsia, cardiac disease).
- Avoid tocolytics in antepartum haemorrhage and abruption.
- Be prepared for increased blood loss from a relaxed uterus.
- Electronic fetal monitoring should be restarted in theatre and maintained as long as possible.
- Avoid maternal hypotension.
  - Uterine blood flow is not subject to autoregulation. Uterine perfusion is therefore correlated with blood pressure. A maternal pressure fall >20 per cent of baseline systolic figure will produce a substantial reduction in uterine perfusion. This will aggravate any acute intrapartum fetal compromise. Thorough evaluation, fluid preloading, patient positioning and drugs can minimize the incidence and degree of hypotension after sympathetic blockage from a spinal or epidural anaesthetic, but it may occur even under the best circumstances. The anaesthetic management can be challenging when acute intrapartum fetal compromise is superimposed on chronic or preexisting fetal compromise. Underlying chronic fetal compromise may be secondary to preeclampsia, hypertension, postmaturity or diabetes. These disorders reduce fetal reserve and the ability to successfully mount a compensatory response to intrapartum hypoxic stress. It is important to avoid even mild hypotension in order to maintain uterine blood flow and placental perfusion in such cases.

Pitfalls

- Failure to change maternal position. (If fetal compromise persists, try right lateral or knee-elbow position because umbilical cord compression rather than aortocaval compression may be the cause).
- Failure to restart FHR monitoring in theatre.
- Routine oxygen administration to the mother.
  - Fetal oxygen saturation depends on placental perfusion rather than maternal oxygen saturation. The promotion and restoration of adequate fetal oxygen delivery should take the form of appropriate maternal positioning, reduction of uterine activity and appropriate intravenous fluid and vasopressor therapy to help ensure adequate uterine blood flow. Supplemental oxygen should be used to improve maternal oxygen saturation as required.
- Failure to communicate within a team may result in undue haste or delays.

References

1. Parer JT, Livingston EG. What is fetal distress? *Am J Obstet Gynecol* 1990;162:1421.

2. Chandraharan E, Arulkumaran S. Prevention of birth asphyxia: responding appropriately to cardiotocograph (CTG) traces. *Best Pract Res Clin Obstet Gynaecol* 2007;21(4):609–24.

3. Maharaj D. Intrapartum fetal resuscitation: a review. *Int J Gynec Obstet* 2007;9(2).

4. Weale NK, Kinsella SM. Intrauterine fetal resuscitation. *Anaesth Intens Care Med* 2007;8:282–5.

5. Kinsella SM, Girgirah K, Scrutton MJL. Rapid sequence spinal for category-1 urgency caesarean section: a case series. *Anaesthesia* 2010;65:664–9.

6. Bogad D, Plaat F. Be wary of awareness – lessons from NAP5 for obstetric anaesthetists. *Int J Obstet Anesth* 2015;24:1–4.

7. Simpson KR. Intrauterine resuscitation during labor: should maternal oxygen administration be a first-line measure? *Semin Fetal Neonatal Med* 2008;13(6):362–7.

8. Dyer RA, Schoeman LK. Fetal distress. In: Ginosar Y, Reynolds F, Halpern S, Weiner C, editors. *Anesthesia and the fetus*. UK: Wiley Blackwell; 2013.

9. Fawole B, Hofmeyr GJ. Maternal oxygen administration for fetal distress. *Cochrane Database Syst Rev* 2012;12:CD000136.

10. Hamel MS, Anderson BL, Rouse DJ. Oxygen for intrauterine resuscitation: of unproved benefit and potentially harmful. *Am J Obstet Gynecol* 2014; 211(2):124–7.

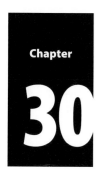

Chapter

30

Medico-legal Issues with CTG

K. Muhunthan and Sabaratnam Arulkumaran

Background

- Cardiotocography refers to the recording of fetal heart rate (FHR) and contractions (tocography).
- Continuous electronic fetal monitoring (EFM) has become a standard practice in high-risk pregnancies and labour in the Western world.
- Despite severely abnormal CTG changes, failure of timely action and nonconsideration of the clinical situation leads to a compromised fetus.
- In-utero fetal death in labour, neonatal death and cerebral palsy associated with abnormal CTGs and asphyxia lead to medical litigation.

Key Facts

Medical negligence involves establishing the causation and liability.

- Presence of abnormal CTG, low Apgar score, low cord arterial pH, assisted ventilation, admission to neonatal intensive care, moderate or severe neonatal encephalopathy and subsequent neurological damage point to asphyxia as a possible cause.
- However, several intrinsic fetal disorders (e.g. severe hypoglycaemia) cause neurological disability, and an abnormal CTG may have been coincidental.
- Causation is best determined by neuroradiologist and paediatric neurologist. The fetus born at term demonstrates certain areas of scarring within the brain on MRI. The thalamus, basal ganglia injury show scarring, reflecting acute profound hypoxia while prolonged partial hypoxia results in bilateral cortical atrophy.[1] Paediatric neurologist supports these findings by demonstrating that the baby has athetoid or dyskinetic cerebral palsy with acute profound hypoxia and spastic quadriplegia with prolonged partial hypoxia.[2]
- Liability is determined by demonstrating that appropriate and timey action was not taken in the presence of an abnormal CTG in that clinical situation.[3]
- Expert opinion is requested to judge whether care provided fell short of what was expected (Bolam principle).[4]

Key Features on the CTG Trace

There are few key CTG patterns that are recognized to be associated with fetal compromise and are described below with example CTGs.[5]

Handbook of CTG Interpretation: From Patterns to Physiology, ed. Edwin Chandraharan. Published by Cambridge University Press. © Cambridge University Press 2017.

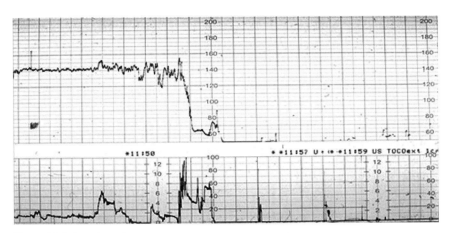

Figure 30.1 Acute hypoxia.

Acute Hypoxia

- Presents with profound deceleration with a heart rate <80 bpm (Figure 30.1).
- The pH can drop on an average by 0.01 per minute.[6,7] The outcome of the fetus/newborn would depend on the physiological reserve of the fetus, actual heart rate (whether it is 40 or 60 bpm), duration of prolonged deceleration before delivery and cause for prolonged deceleration (e.g. abruption placentae, cord prolapse or scar rupture).
- An example of prolonged deceleration or bradycardia is given below. If prolonged, it can cause fetal death, or if born asphyxiated, it may lead to neurological injury associated with acute profound hypoxia.
- The thalamus and basal ganglia region gets affected and leads to athetoid or dyskinetic type of cerebral palsy.
- An example of such a trace is shown in Figure 30.1.

Subacute Hypoxia

- Presents with prolonged decelerations (Figure 30.2).
- The FHR is below baseline rate for a longer time (e.g. >60 to 90 seconds) than at baseline rate (<30 seconds).[8]
- With such FHR, there is less than optimal circulation through the placenta over a given time, especially if the FHR drops to <80 bpm. With such a trace (Figure 30.2), some of the fetuses would get compromised with the progression of acidosis of approximately 0.01 every 2–3 minutes.

Gradually Developing Hypoxia

The CTG trace usually starts with a normal baseline rate, normal baseline variability, accelerations and no decelerations.

Once decelerations start due to cord compression (variable decelerations) or reduced placental reserve (late decelerations), hypoxia can set in leading to catecholamine surge and rise in the baseline rate.

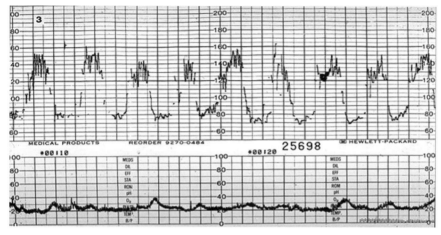

Figure 30.2 Subacute hypoxia.

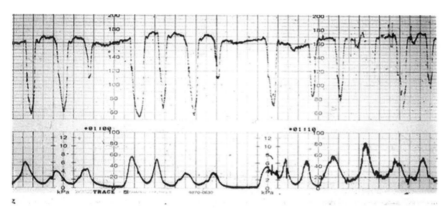

Figure 30.3 Gradually evolving hypoxia with loss of baseline variability.

With increasing hypoxia, accelerations do not appear and decelerations get deeper and wider (i.e. longer duration).

The FHR reaches a peak rate beyond which it is unable to increase the FHR. Even with this rate, if oxygenation to the autonomic system cannot be maintained, the baseline variability tends to get gradually reduced to almost flat baseline variability (Figure 30.3).

In the presence of normal baseline variability, 97 percent of the times the pH is likely to be >7.0.[9]

When acidosis gets worse, within a short period the heart rate comes down and becomes asystolic and may end as a stillbirth.

If delivered at the 'peak' heart rate after 1 to 2 hours of the FHR baseline variability becoming 'flat' ('distress platform'), the baby may be born asphyxiated (hypoxia in the tissues and metabolic acidosis) and may suffer neurological injury or bilateral cortical injury leading to cerebral palsy with spastic quadriparesis due to prolonged partial hypoxia.[1]

Figure 30.3 gives an example of gradually developing hypoxia that has gone into the stage of possible acidosis that may lead to an asphyxiated baby.

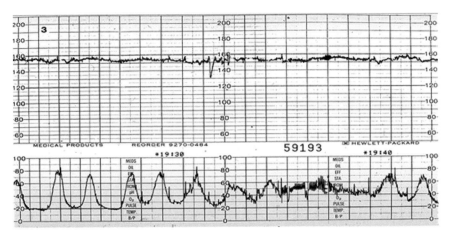

Figure 30.4 Chronic or long-standing hypoxia.

Long-standing or Preexisting Hypoxia

- A fetus that is hypoxic and with early evidence of acidosis may show a nonreactive trace (no accelerations) with absent or markedly reduced baseline variability and shallow decelerations (blunted CNS response) to hypoxic stress produced by contractions.
- A fetus with such a trace may withstand the stress of contractions for variable number of hours without any change on the CTG trace before the fetus gets severely acidotic and has a cardiovascular collapse.
- Such a trace is shown in Figure 30.4. If delivered earlier, the fetus would be in a better condition.
- Not all the fetuses may be neurologically affected, and with such a trace, earlier the delivery better the outcome.
- Figure 30.4 is an example of a CTG trace where the fetus may be already acidotic.

Anaemia and Sinusoidal CTG Trace

Causes could be:[10]

- Physiological – sucking the thumb, smacking its lips – as demonstrated by ultrasound examination.
- Pathological – a severe anaemia causes a sinusoidal pattern although the mechanism is not known.

Causes for fetal anaemia:

- Rhesus sensitization, Kell, Duff antibodies
- ABO antibodies give rise to neonatal jaundice, not fetal anaemia
- Lewis a and b and M and N antibodies usually do not cause fetal anaemia.
- Parvo virus infection.
- Fetomaternal transfusion.
- Vasa praevia and bleeding due to the rupture of vessels.
- Alpha thalassemia.

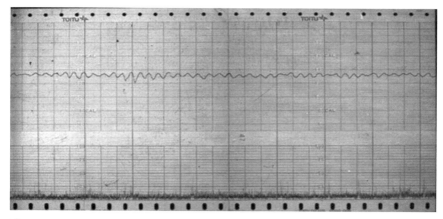

Figure 30.5 Typical sinusoidal trace secondary to chronic fetal anaemia.

Key Pathophysiology behind Patterns Seen on the CTG Trace

- Acute hypoxia is due to reversible (hypotension due to epidural, vaginal examination, artificial rupture of membranes and, at times, no cause may be identified) and nonreversible causes (abruption, cord prolapse, scar rupture). To maintain normal blood gases and pH, the FHR may be at 140 bpm, i.e. 1,400 circulations through the placenta per minute. When the FHR is 80 bpm, there are only 800 circulations through the placenta, i.e. misses 600 circulations. This causes a marked reduction in CO_2 expulsion and accumulation in the fetus and respiratory acidosis, and in addition, the reduction in oxygen intake promotes anaerobic metabolism and metabolic acidosis. Hence the drop of pH is approximately 0.01 per minute. In addition, there is impact of coronary filling as well.
- Subacute hypoxia is usually due to intermittent prolonged cord compression that may be exaggerated by oxytocin infusion or posture. The more the FHR is below baseline FHR and the lower the FHR, the higher is the lack of oxygen intake and expulsion of CO_2, i.e. suboptimal circulation which leads to build up of acidosis.
- Gradually developing hypoxia is due to ongoing cord compression interfering with umbilical cord flow (variable decelerations) or due to a reduction of retroplacental blood flow (late decelerations). With gradual reduction of oxygen and hypoxia, there is catecholamine surge that increases baseline FHR and peripheral vasoconstriction. Despite the increase in FHR, if there is time taken for coronary filling is inadequate, then decelerations become deeper and of longer duration. A further reduction of oxygen to the fetus affects the autonomic system resulting in a marked reduction in baseline variability.
- Long-standing hypoxia is due to nonrecognized intrauterine growth restriction, infection, prolonged pregnancy, placental malfunction (i.e. usually placental insufficiency). The central nervous system may be under the influence of hypoxia, thus resulting in blunted response and shallow decelerations. Additional contractions would cause further acidosis and sudden bradycardia and collapse.
- A sinusoidal pattern of concern is due to fetal anaemia. The exact mechanism by which anaemia produces a sinusoidal pattern is not known. It is believed to be due to acidosis to the brain centres.

Recommended Management

- In acute hypoxia, the 3, 6, 9, 12, 15 rule is useful.[11] Three minutes of low FHR makes it a CTG of concern. If it is due to irreversible causes of abruption, cord prolapse or scar rupture, steps should be taken for immediate delivery. If the CTG is abnormal prior to bradycardia/prolonged deceleration or if there is evidence of clinical compromise (e.g. IUGR, thick meconium), steps for delivery should be taken by 6 minutes and in others by 9 minutes if conservative measures of postural change, stopping oxytocin and tocolytics when needed do not reverse bradycardia/prolonged deceleration. Earlier the delivery, better the condition and aim for delivery within 15 to 30 minutes.
- In subacute hypoxia, conservative measures of change of posture, hydration, stopping oxytocin and tocolytics should be considered as needed, but if the FHR does not return to near normality, operative delivery is advised unless spontaneous vaginal delivery is imminent. Caesarean or instrumental delivery should be undertaken depending on the stage of labour within 30 to 40 minutes.[12]
- In gradually developing hypoxia, delivery should be undertaken when there is maximal rise in baseline rate with increasing depth and duration of decelerations with reduction of interdeceleration intervals and marked reduction in baseline variability for a period of 1 hour unless fetal scalp pH shows that further observation is safe.
- In long-standing hypoxic patterns, early delivery (40–60 minutes) should be undertaken in the presence of significant meconium, absence of fetal movements, bleeding per vagina, IUGR or prolonged pregnancy. In the absence of such symptoms, observation could be continued for up to 90 minutes before consideration of delivery.
- In sinusoidal patterns, if fetal anaemia is suspected by blood group antibody testing, Kelihauer–Betke test for fetomaternal transfusion, or increased blood flow velocity of fetal middle cerebral artery, then delivery should be undertaken. In addition to sinusoidal, if late decelerations are present with contractions, early delivery is advised.

Key Tips to Optimize Management

- Better understanding of the significance of CTG patterns based on pathophysiology (attending master classes, appropriate e-learning programs, books, in-hospital case reviews with CTG).
- CTG is an investigation, and hence management decision should be based on the clinical situation in addition to CTG.
- Requesting a senior person to review CTGs when in doubt.
- Central monitoring systems that help other people also to observe the CTG ('neighbourhood watch') and discuss it with the caregiver.
- Where possible and appropriate to use adjunct methods – fetal ECG (STAN monitoring) or fetal scalp blood sampling (FBS) for pH or lactate.
- Appropriate and timely intervention when conservative measures do not reverse the CTG pattern.
- Adequate staffing including senior staff and ready availability of theatre facilities.

Pitfalls

Based on the Fourth Confidential Enquiry into Stillbirths and Deaths in Infancy (CESDI) and reports from the National Health Services Litigations Authority (NHSLA),[13,14] the common pitfalls are:

- Inability to interpret the CTG trace
- Failure to incorporate the clinical picture
- Delay in taking action
- Poor communication between team members

Failure to incorporate the clinical feature can be due either to a preexisting situation making the fetus at risk where acidosis can develop faster with an abnormal CTG compared to an appropriately grown fetus at term with clear liquor or to injudicious management that puts the fetus at risk. They are listed below:

Fetus at Risk

- Preterm
- Postterm
- Intrauterine growth restriction
- Thick meconium with scanty fluid
- Intrauterine infection
- Intrapartum bleeding

Fetus at Possible Risk Due to Injudicious Management

- Injudicious use of oxytocin
- Epidural in advanced labour and with a CTG showing abnormal pattern
- Difficult instrumental delivery, shoulder dystocia, vaginal breech delivery
- Acute events (cord prolapse, abruption, scar rupture)
- Suspicious/abnormal admission FHR on CTG or auscultation

Consequences of Mismanagement

Mismanagement leads to a situation from normoxaemia to hypoxaemia (lack of oxygen in blood) to hypoxia (lack of oxygen in tissue) and asphyxia (lack of oxygen in tissue and metabolic acidosis).

Hypoxia and metabolic acidosis leads to cell dysfunction in various tissues and may present as:

1. Heart failure
2. Pneumocytes type 2 injury lead to less surfactant factor
3. GI system 'necrotizing enterocolitis'
4. Renal failure
5. Endothelial damage leads to DIC (disseminated intravascular coagulation)
6. CNS – cerebral oedema, seizures or coma (grades II and III neonatal encephalopathy). Cell death could lead to cerebral palsy.
7. Stillbirth or neonatal death

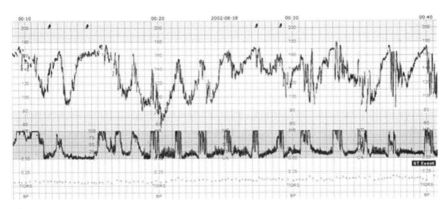

Figure 30.6

- Needless to say, mismanagement leads to medical litigation. Litigation can also be an unpleasant experience and have significant long-term consequences for the working lives for healthcare staff involved.
- Escalating costs of claims and insurance premiums have led to a major concern for maternity service providers across most of the countries.[14]
- Malpractice fears are also believed to have contributed, in small part, to the rising defensive practice in obstetrics.[15]
- Anyhow, most malpractice claims seem to be unrelated to the incompetence of an individual provider but to systemic failures that overwhelm competent people working in a highly imperfect and complex environment.
- Report published by NHSLA in October 2012 provides an analysis of the various clinical situations that have led to maternity claims. In a 10-year analysis of maternity claims (between 1 April 2000 and 31 March 2010), there were 5,087 claims with a total value of £3.1 billion.[14]
- This amounts to <0.1 percent of births, indicating that the vast majority of births do not result in a clinical negligence claim.

Exercise

A 28-year-old gravida 2 is in spontaneous normal labour. She has no high-risk factors and she is in the active second stage of labour. She was monitored for audible abnormality of the FHR. Abdominally the fetus was estimated to be 3.8 kg and the head was 0/5th palpable. Vaginally there was clear amniotic fluid, she was fully dilated, and the occiput was in left occipito transverse position at station 0 to +1. There is ++ caput and ++ moulding. The CTG trace is shown in Figure 30.6.

1. Describe your plan of action.
   a. Observe for another hour
   b. Perform FBS
   c. Perform caesarean section
   d. Perform instrumental delivery
   e. Give acute tocolysis and await further descent

References

1. Myers RE. Four patterns of perinatal brain damage and the conditions of occurrence in primates. *Advances in neurology. Vol. X.* Eds. BS Meldrum and CD Marsden. Raven Press, New York. 1975; pp. 223–34.

2. MacLennan A. A template for defining a causal relation between acute intrapartum events and cerebral palsy: international consensus statement. *BMJ* 1999;319:1054–9.

3. Williams B, Arulkumaran S. Cardiotocography and medico-legal issues. *Best Pract Res Clin Obstet Gynaecol* 2004;18(3):457–66.

4. Electronic fetal monitoring: medico-legal issues. *Fetal monitoring in practice.* Second edition. Eds. G Donald and S Arulkumaran. Butterworth Heinemann, Oxford. 2008; pp. 225–9.

5. Arulkumaran S. Fetal surveillance in labour. *Munro Kerr's operative obstetrics.* Twelfth edition. Eds. TF Baskett, AA Calder and S Arulkumaran. Saunders Elsevier, Ediburgh. 2014; pp. 41–56.

6. Ingemarsson I, Arulkumaran S, Ratnam SS. Single injection of terbutaline in term labor. Effect on fetal pH in cases with prolonged bradycardia. *Am J Obstet Gynecol* 1985;153:859–65.

7. Leung TY, Chung PW, Rogers MS, et al. Urgent caesarean delivery for fetal bradycardia. *Obstet Gynecol* 2009;114(5):1023–8.

8. Cahill AG, Kimberly AR, Odibo AO, Maconaes GA. Association and prediction of neonatal acidaemia. *Am J Obstet Gynecol* 2012;207:206–8.

9. Williams KP, Galerneau F. Intrapartum fetal heart rate patterns in the prediction of neonatal acidemia. *Am J Obstet Gynecol* 2003;188:820–3.

10. Cardiotocographic interpretation: more difficult problems. Sinusoidal pattern. *Fetal monitoring in practice.* Third edition. Eds. G Donald and S Arulkumaran. Butterworth Heinemann, Oxford. 2008; pp. 159–88.

11. Intrapartum care. Care of healthy women and their babies during childbirth. NICE clinical guideline 190, December 2014, pp 39–57.

12. The role of scal pH. *Fetal monitoring in practice.* Third edition. Eds. G Donald and S Arulkumaran. Butterworth Heinemann, Oxford. 2008; pp. 189–203.

13. Confidential enquiry into stillbirths and deaths in infancy. Fourth annual report. 1997. Maternal and Child Health Research Consortium.

14. Ten years of maternity claims. An analysis of NHS Litigation Authority data. NHS Litigation Authority. October 2012.

15. Schifrin BS, Cohen WR. The effect of malpractice claims on the use of caesarean section. *Best Pract Res Clin Obstet Gynaecol* 2012:S1521-6934(12)00165-4.

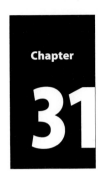

Chapter

31

Ensuring Competency in Intrapartum Fetal Monitoring
The Role of GIMS

Virginia Lowe and Edwin Chandraharan

Background

St George's Maternity Unit employs CTG and fetal ECG (ST-Analyser or STAN) to assess fetal well-being during labour. Both these tests require clinicians to have sufficient knowledge and expertise in order to recognize and correctly interpret common CTG changes. To understand the importance of these changes requires an understanding of the pathophysiology of FHR control and hypoxia, and, additionally, the knowledge of associated clinical circumstances is essential in order to ensure appropriate management. The 'Confidential Enquiry into Stillbirths and Deaths in Infancy' report in the mid-1990s concluded that 50 per cent of intrapartum-related deaths could have been prevented if the clinicians involved had instituted alternative management. Lack of knowledge regarding CTG interpretation was identified as a significant factor within the report, as well as failure to incorporate the whole clinical picture, incorrect or delayed action and communication/common sense issues. The Chief Medical Officer's report 'Intrapartum-Related Deaths: 500 Missed Opportunities' in 2007 has also highlighted the above issues as recurring themes in obstetric care.

St George's Intrapartum Monitoring Strategy (GIMS) comprises intensive, physiology-based CTG training, use of fetal ECG (STAN) to reduce the false-positive rate of CTG and a mandatory competency testing for all midwives and obstetricians. This combination aims to deepen the appreciation clinicians have for the intricacies of fetal monitoring and promotes consistency across the service.

Objectives

1. To ensure that *all* staff (midwives and obstetricians – trainees, middle-grade doctors and consultants) who interpret CTG/STAN traces are comprehensively trained.
2. To ensure that all staff continuously update their knowledge and skills in fetal monitoring.
3. To ensure competency in CTG/STAN interpretation by providing training as well as conducting an assessment process.
4. To provide support to staff who do not perform up to 85 per cent competency in CTG/STAN interpretation to maintain a high standard of care.

Strategies

Intense Physiology-Based CTG Training

This involves a deeper understanding of fetal pathophysiology: instead of morphologically classifying decelerations as 'early', 'variable' and 'late', the underlying mechanism is explored (e.g. baroreceptor- or chemoreceptor-mediated) as well as the fetal response to ongoing hypoxic or mechanical stresses. In addition, education focusses on the consideration of the features of the type of intrapartum (acute, subacute or a gradually evolving) or chronic (long-standing) fetal hypoxia on the CTG trace and encourages differentiation of a compensatory fetal response from decompensation. Case scenarios are discussed in depth to reinforce the importance of considering the whole clinical picture and to embed learning points.

Use of Fetal ECG (STAN)

Fetal ECG is used to determine the energy balance within a central organ (myocardium) so as to identify the onset of myocardial glycogenolysis as a mechanism to maintain energy balance with the onset of anaerobic metabolism. This may help reduce the false-positive rate of CTG while improving perinatal outcomes. See Chapter 22.

Competency Testing

The assessment tool comprises questions on 'pattern recognition' as determined by current guidelines on intrapartum FHR monitoring; knowledge of fetal pathophysiology including the types of hypoxia; questions on situational awareness and considering the wider clinical picture (e.g. recognition of features of MHR, injudicious use of syntocinon etc.). There is an agreed policy within the unit which summarizes the expectations, an extract of which is shown below:

Training and Assessment

a. New Staff

All new staff (midwives and all grades of obstetricians involved in intrapartum fetal monitoring) will be provided CTG/STAN training as part of their induction. After their training, they will be required to obtain 85 per cent competency in assessment in both CTG as well as STAN to demonstrate their knowledge in intrapartum fetal monitoring.

Obstetricians are required to attend weekly CTG meetings, which are held on Tuesdays and Fridays, to update their knowledge and skills in CTG/STAN interpretation. It is recommended that they attend at least two such meetings every month. Minimum requirements would be to attend CTG Meetings at least once a month and to attend at least 12 meetings in 6 months or to complete the online CTG Assessment Tool at least twice in 6 months. Midwives are strongly encouraged to attend as often as shift pattern permits.

b. Existing Staff

All staff are expected to undergo a formal CTG Training (minimum 3 hours) once every 12 months, in addition to attending the CTG Meetings as stated earlier.

All staff who have passed the assessments in CTG/STAN will be required to re-sit the test at least once every two years, or earlier, if required (for example if they are involved in two or more adverse incidents which involved failures in CTG/STAN interpretation or they have been involved

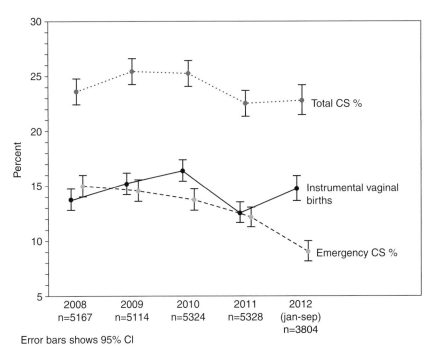

Error bars shows 95% CI

Figure 31.1 Trends in total and emergency caesarean section rates.

with an SI where failure to interpret CTG/STAN by the clinician concerned contributed to the poor outcome).

Outcomes

The approach to intrapartum FHR monitoring has resulted in a significant reduction in intrapartum emergency section rate from 15 per cent in 2008 to 8 per cent in 2012 (Figure 31.1). Despite commencing a regional service for morbidly adherent placentae and a regional bariatric service, both of which may increase the total caesarean section rate, currently the emergency caesarean section rate remains between 6.1 and 8.2 per cent. The neonatal metabolic acidosis rate as well as the HIE rates have also halved during this period (Figure 31.2), and currently, the maternity unit has half the nationally reported HIE rate in the United Kingdom.

Discussion

CTG interpretation that relies on 'pattern recognition' is fraught with inter- and intra-observer variability, leading to overdiagnosis as well as failure to recognize features of ongoing intrapartum hypoxia. These errors may lead to unnecessary intrapartum operative interventions and hypoxic-ischaemic injury, respectively. The St George's approach to intrapartum FHR monitoring focusses on fetal physiology and a deeper understanding of the features observed on the CTG trace so as to avoid flaws of 'pattern recognition' and has resulted in halving of intrapartum caesarean section and adverse perinatal outcome rates. This training is facilitated by a group of clinicians with a particular interest in fetal monitoring, including midwives employed as CTG specialists who maintain competency records

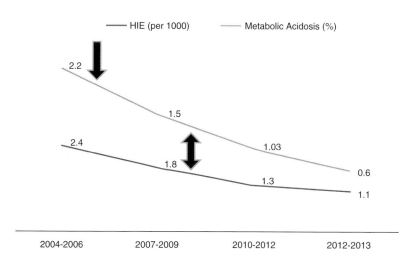

Trends in Neonatal Metabolic Acidosis and HIE

—— HIE (per 1000)   —— Metabolic Acidosis (%)

2.2

1.5

2.4

1.03

1.8

1.3

0.6

1.1

2004-2006   2007-2009   2010-2012   2012-2013

Arrow- Commencement of Intense training on Fetal Physiology
Double Arrow- Introduction of Mandatory Competency Testing

Figure 31.2 Rates of neonatal metabolic acidosis rate and HIE rate.

and can be available for one-to-one support. Introducing mandatory competency testing is not without its challenges: there can be a level of anxiety around the formal assessment process, and a clear pathway is required where competency is not achieved in order to maintain patient safety. These issues are mitigated by ensuring all clinicians involved in CTG training maintain a strong clinical presence and, therefore, are in a position to take advantage of educational opportunities in practice and provide consistent support while also maintaining credibility and an appreciation of the challenges faced by frontline staff. Where clinically appropriate, STAN is routinely employed as a 'central organ test' to reduce the false-positive rate of CTG. Although meta-analysis has not reported any significant decrease in caesarean section rates and gives conflicting information about reduction in neonatal metabolic acidosis, data from St George shows that the use of STAN in combination with an intensive physiology-based CTG training and mandatory competency testing may result in significant improvement in perinatal outcomes while reducing unnecessary intrapartum operative interventions.

Conclusion

All maternity units should consider training midwives and obstetricians in fetal physiology so as to critically analyse the pathophysiological mechanisms behind the features observed on the CTG trace. This may avoid errors due to inter- and intra-observer variations secondary to merely relying on 'pattern recognition' based on existing guidelines. This training should be followed up by mandatory competency testing on CTG interpretation. Once the staff are fully trained in fetal pathophysiology, the use of STAN appears to significantly reduce intrapartum emergency caesarean section rates and improve perinatal outcomes (neonatal metabolic acidosis and HIE rates).

Further Reading

1. Ayres-de-Campos D, Arteiro D, Costa-Santos C, et al. Knowledge of adverse neonatal outcome alters clinicians' interpretation of the intrapartum cardiotocograph. *BJOG* 2011;118(8):978e84.

2. Nurani R, Chandraharan E, Lowe V, et al. Misidentification of maternal heart rate as fetal on cardiotocography during the second stage of labor: the role of the fetal electrocardiograph. *Acta Obstet Gynecol Scan* 2012;91(12):1428e32.

3. McDonnell S, Chandraharan E. The pathophysiology of CTGs and types of intrapartum hypoxia. *Curr Wom Health Rev* 2013;9:158e68.

4. Chandraharan E, Lowe V, Arulkumaran S. Pathological decelerations on CTG: time for FPS or FBS? *Int J Obstet Gynecol* 2012:S309.

5. Chandraharan E, Arulkumaran S. Prevention of birth asphyxia: responding appropriately to cardiotocograph (CTG) traces. *Best Pract Res Clin Obstet Gynaecol* 2007;21(4):609e24.

6. Chandraharan E, Lowe V, Ugwumadu A, Arulkumaran S. Impact of fetal ECG (STAN) and competency based training on intrapartum interventions and perinatal outcomes at a teaching hospital in London: 5 year analysis. *BJOG* 2013;120(s1):428–429.

7. Pinas A, Chandraharan E. Continuous cardiotocography during labour: analysis, classification and management. *Best Pract Res Clin Obstet Gynaecol* 2015;25:S1521-6934.

8. Chandraharan E, Lowe V, Penna L, Ugwumadu A, Arulkumaran S. Does 'process based' training in fetal monitoring improve knowledge of cardiotocograph (CTG) among midwives and obstetricians? *Book of Abstracts.* Ninth RCOG International Scientific Meeting, Athens, 2011. www.rcog.org.uk/events/rcog-congresses/athens-2011

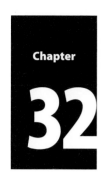

Chapter 32

Physiology-Based CTG Training

Does It Really Matter?

Sara Ledger and Edwin Chandraharan

Key Facts

Baby Lifeline's Role in CTG Training

Baby Lifeline is a unique, UK-based mother-and-baby charity that was established in 1981 after its founder tragically lost three premature babies successively. Its mission is to ensure the healthiest outcome possible in pregnancy and birth; it does this by developing evidence-based, highly relevant, vital training for multidisciplinary teams working in the maternity sector. Course topics and content are chosen based on recommendations from confidential enquiries and pertinent reports highlighting key areas of suboptimal care within the maternity sector. The Charity was established in 1981 and started its important relationship with multidisciplinary training in 1999, following on from recommendations from the Confidential Enquiry into Stillbirths and Deaths' (CESDI) fourth annual report.[1]

Centres and Delegates

Baby Lifeline staged its first CTG masterclass in 2005, and demand has increased each year, with a total of 10 one-day courses and one two-day course being held in 2015 at multiple centres across the United Kingdom and Channel Islands. Baby Lifeline has staged a total of 42 physiology-based CTG study-days since 2005 in 27 different centres. Over 1,840 multiprofessional delegates (79 per cent midwives, 16 per cent obstetricians, 5 per cent legal professionals) have attended masterclasses from a diverse range of maternity units and organizations within the United Kingdom and internationally.

Structure and Aim of Masterclass

The structure of the courses consists of 1-day ('CTG Master Class: Fundamentals of Fetal Monitoring') and two-day courses ('CTG Master Class: A Deeper Understanding') with postcourse materials to cement knowledge and enable delegates to carry out vital, evidence-based modifications to practice.

The aim of the masterclass is to provide evidence-based training on CTG interpretation based on fetal physiology and pathophysiology of intrapartum hypoxic injury so as to reduce hypoxic-ischaemic encephalopathy while reducing unnecessary operative interventions. Delegates are invited to engage with CTG traces and thought-provoking research and look reflectively at their own practice, centred on logical physiology-based reasoning.

Handbook of CTG Interpretation: From Patterns to Physiology, ed. Edwin Chandraharan. Published by Cambridge University Press. © Cambridge University Press 2017.

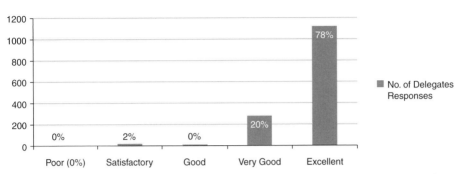

Figure 32.1 A graph to show postcourse delegates' responses regarding overall quality of education of both 1-day and 2-day CTG masterclass (2005–2015).

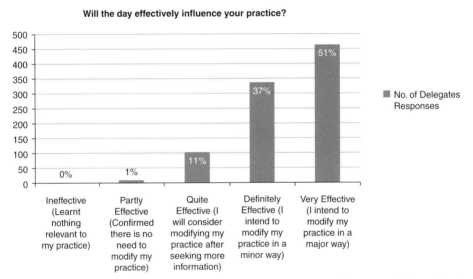

Figure 32.2 A graph to show postcourse delegates' responses regarding the effectiveness of 1-day and 2-day CTG masterclasses at influencing practice.

Key Outcomes

Delegate Feedback

Structural feedback has been excellent, with 98 per cent of delegates reporting that the quality of education was 'Very Good' (20 per cent) or 'Excellent' (78 per cent) (Figure 32.1). Interestingly, Figure 32.2 illustrates that, of the 914 delegates that responded following the course, only 10 (1 per cent) felt that the study-day confirmed that there was no need to modify their practice. The remaining 99 per cent reported that they intended to modify practice in a minor or major way (88 per cent), or they would consider modifying their practice after

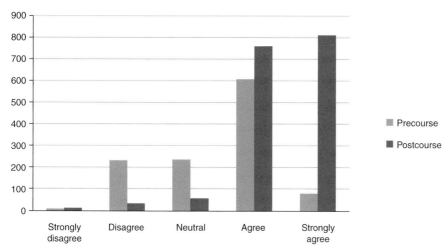

Figure 32.3 A graph to show how many delegates agreed or disagreed with statements relating to how confident they felt about course objectives precourse and postcourse.

seeking more information (11 per cent). The majority of respondent delegates (51 per cent) intended to modify their practice in a *major way* following the course.

Anonymised delegate responses to statements relating to key course objectives also infer that the CTG masterclass would have an effective influence on practice. Delegate confidence in knowledge was quantitatively measured by using a five-point Likert scale ranging from 'Strongly Disagree' to 'Strongly Agree' to the statements below:

I understand the control of fetal heart rate and the factors that affect the features observed on the Cardiotocograph (CTG).

I understand the types of intrapartum hypoxia and resultant features observed on the CTG Trace.

I appreciate the wider clinical picture; such as, inflammation, infection and meconium whilst interpreting CTG Traces.

I feel confident in my application of National Guidelines and additional tests of fetal well-being.

I feel confident in my recognition of processes whilst interpreting CTG Traces.

The variance in responses pre- and postcourse showed an increase in confidence postcourse. On average, across all statements and delegates that completed the tests, an increase of 35 per cent delegates reportedly 'agreed' or 'strongly agreed' with the preceding statements than prior to the course. A total of 94 per cent 'agreed' or 'strongly agreed' that they were confident and understood the key knowledge points postcourse, as opposed to 59 per cent prior to the course (Figure 32.3).

Increased confidence in technical skills inevitably promotes shared learning of evidence-based practice on labour wards and could lead to increased patient safety.

"This has been an excellent day. I feel totally inspired. I hope to instigate positive changes to my practice and, as a team leader, that of others."

"This is an excellent course. I have learned more today than in 16 years of training. I will try and constitute this management in my unit."

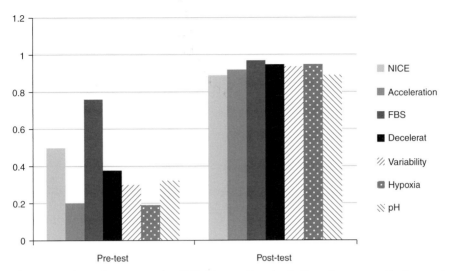

Figure 32.4 Pre- and post-test results of 810 delegates. Note the significant improvement in all parameters tested after training.

One of the best study days I have attended. Qualified in 1977! (2014)

I found the course extremely interesting, motivating and empowering … I now feel far more confident in my knowledge of physiology, therefore more confident in my interpretation. (2014)

Impact of Training: Pre- and Post-Tests

Eight hundred and ten midwives and obstetricians underwent 10 questions on NICE guidelines, type of intrapartum hypoxia, fetal response to stress as well as decision making (e.g. performing fetal blood sampling or operative interventions) before the commencement of the CTG masterclass (the 'Pre-Test'). They answered the same questions after 8 hours of intense, physiology-based CTG training (the 'Post-Test'). Figure 32.4 shows significant improvement in the knowledge of NICE guidelines, understanding of the types of hypoxia, fetal response as well as on decision making. This illustrates the positive impact of physiology-based CTG training on improving knowledge and decision making among midwives and obstetricians.

Key Challenges to Multiprofessional Training in Physiology-Based CTG Interpretation

Many reports and national bodies have recommended that improvements to training would lead to improvements in safety and outcomes.[1-4] However, despite these recommendations, investment in external CPD (continuous professional development) courses appears to be insufficient. A recent survey was completed by delegates that attended Baby Lifeline's training in the first half of 2014; it showed that 59 per cent of delegates had to self-fund the cost of attending courses, including travel and accommodation, or were given a fully funded or part-funded place by Baby Lifeline (Figure 32.5). An additional 5 per cent of delegates conveyed that places were paid for by Royal Colleges or unions ('other'). Just 38 per cent of delegates reported that they were supported by their organization to attend the training, 2 per cent of which were legal professionals.

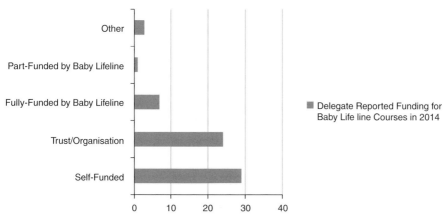

Figure 32.5 A graph to show how delegates self-reportedly paid for Baby Lifeline study-day places in the first half of 2014. The graph shows the percentage of responses for each answer.

These findings support a report published by The King's Fund in 2008, which investigated healthcare professionals' views about safety in maternity services. In the short questionnaire, clinicians reported a 'general feeling that there are insufficient funds for CPD',[5] with many of the direct quotes communicating a great degree of familiarity:

> Midwives should have paid time away from their work environment to reflect on practice and learn from difficult situations. They should not be expected to study in their annual leave and to pay for this study time. (Midwife/independent midwife, 3–10 years' experience) (p.15)

In order to alleviate some of the financial pressures on both self-funding delegates and financially crippled NHS organizations, Baby Lifeline gained support from sympathetic law firms, leading training equipment manufacturers and voluntary expert faculty; this enabled Baby Lifeline to offer study-days at subsidized rates to all delegates, which is in fact 75 per cent less than the course fee of some professional bodies that conduct CTG courses in the United Kingdom. Despite low costs for training and some fully funded places, delegate attendance was lower than anticipated in 2014. CTG masterclasses with delegate numbers as low as 18 were delivered in some regions of the United Kingdom. This is likely to reflect the staffing pressures experienced by many maternity units and the inability of staff to get time off to attend training.

Patterns in the structural differences of Baby Lifeline's CTG courses (1 day and 2 days) may also reflect an adjusted culture due to underresourced maternity units and, consequently, limited study leave. From 2011 to 2012, 80 per cent of CTG masterclasses staged by Baby Lifeline were the 2-day masterclasses; however, this fell to 17 per cent from 2013 to 2015.

Another key challenge for physiology-based CTG training is the current guideline on CTG interpretation which has been published by the National Institute of Health and Care Excellence (NICE), is based on pattern recognition. It is quite alarming that even 5 years after the publication of NICE guidelines on CTG interpretation in 2007,[6] <50 per cent of delegates answered questions on NICE guidelines correctly (Figure 32.4). This illustrates the flaws of using 'pattern recognition' as it causes confusion among midwives and obstetricians and leads to errors in the classification of CTG traces.

The most recent updated version of this guideline (December 2014) not only had used even more confusing terminology, very unfortunately, several of its recommendations were not based on robust scientific evidence but on the personal clinical experience of three obstetricians on the Guideline Development Group.[7] This is likely to create confusion and worsen outcomes for women and their babies in the future. In fact, a National Survey of Labour Ward Lead Obstetricians in the United Kingdom, which was presented at the National Labour Ward Leads' Meeting in March 2015 at the Royal College of Obstetricians and Gynaecologists, confirmed that more than half of the consultant obstetricians (labour ward leads) surveyed felt that the updated NICE guidelines on CTG interpretation would worsen communication in the labour ward, increase operative interventions and also may increase the incidence of hypoxic-ischaemic encephalopathy. Therefore, clinicians should be cautious in implementing non–evidence-based guidelines on CTG interpretation, if it is felt that they may in fact worsen perinatal outcomes and make communication in the labour ward difficult. Instead, a physiology-based CTG interpretation may help improve neonatal outcomes while avoiding unnecessary operative interventions.[8,9]

Conclusion

Baby Lifeline has conducted a total of 42 physiology-based CTG study-days since 2005 in 27 different centres, and over 1,840 multiprofessional delegates (79 per cent midwives, 16 per cent obstetricians, 5 per cent legal professionals) have attended these 'CTG masterclasses' so far. However, despite these courses being subsidized, funding by cash-strapped NHS maternity units and staffing issues pose a major challenge. However, it has been clearly shown that the use of 'physiology-based CTG training', mandatory competency and a test of central organ oxygenation (fetal ECG or STAN) reduces intrapartum emergency caesarean sections and rates of hypoxic-ischaemic encephalopathy.[8,9] Therefore, continued investment in physiology-based CTG interpretation is essential to avoid hypoxic-ischaemic brain injury and its sequelae as well as unnecessary intrapartum operative interventions.

References

1. Maternal and Child Health Research Consortium. (1997). *Confidential Enquiry into Stillbirths and Deaths in Infancy: 4th Annual Report*. London: Maternal and Child Health Research Consortium.

2. NHS Litigation Authority. (2012). *Ten Years of Maternity Claims: An Analysis of NHS Litigation Authority Data*. London: NHS Litigation Authority.

3. Royal College of Gynaecologists. (1999). *Towards Safer Childbirth: Minimum Standards for the Organisation of Labour Wards*. London: RCOG Press.

4. Royal College of Obstetricians and Gynaecologists (2007). *Safer Childbirth: Minimum Standards for the Organisation and Delivery of Care in Labour*. London: RCOG Press.

5. Smith, A., Dixon, A. (2008). Health care professionals' views about safety in maternity services. The King's Fund.

6. *Intrapartum care: care of healthy women and their babies during childbirth*. NICE guideline number 55. 2007.

7. *Intrapartum care: care of healthy women and their babies during childbirth*. NICE guideline number CG 190. December 2014.

8. Chandraharan E, Lowe V, Ugwumadu A, Arulkumaran S. Impact of fetal ECG (STAN) and competency based training on intrapartum interventions and perinatal outcomes at a teaching hospital

in London: 5 year analysis. *BJOG*. 2013; 120(s1):428–429.

9. Chandraharan E, Lowe V, Penna L, Ugwumadu A, Arulkumaran S. Does 'process based' training in fetal monitoring improve knowledge of cardiotocograph (CTG) among midwives and obstetricians? *Book of Abstracts*. Ninth RCOG International Scientific Meeting, Athens, 2011. www.rcog.org.uk/events/rcog-congresses/athens-2011.

Appendix

Rational Use of FIGO Guidelines in Clinical Practice

The International Federation of Gynecology and Obstetrics (FIGO) released its revised guidelines on CTG in October 2015 in collaboration with 37 member societies and with a consensus panel comprising of 50 CTG experts around the world.

Table A1 CTG Classification Criteria, Interpretation and Recommended Management

	Normal	Suspicious	Pathological
Baseline	110–160	Lacking at leastonecharacteristic ofnormality, but with nopathological features	<100 bpm
Variability	5–25		Reduced variability for > 50 min, increased variability for >30 min, or sinusoidal pattern for > 30 min
Decelerations	No repetitive* decelerations		Repetitive* late or prolonged decelerations during >30 min or 20 min if reduced variability, or one prolonged deceleration >5 min
Interpretation	Fetus with no hypoxia/acidosis	Fetus with a low probability of having hypoxia/acidosis	Fetus with a high probability of having hypoxia/acidosis
Clinical management	No intervention necessary to improve fetal oxygenation state	Action to correct reversible causes if identified, close monitoring or additional methods to evaluate fetal oxygenation	Immediate action to correct reversible causes, additional methods to evaluate fetal oxygenation (Chapter 4), or if this is not posible, expedite delivery; in acute situations (cord prolapse, uterine rupture or placental abruption), immediate delivery should be accomplished

The presence of accelerations denotes a fetus that does not have hypoxia/acidosis, but their absence during labour is of uncertain significance.

*Decelerations are repetitive in nature when they are associated with >50 percent of uterine contractions.

Clinical Decision

Several factors, including gestational age and medication administered to the mother, can affect FHR features, so CTG analysis needs to be integrated with other clinical information for a comprehensive interpretation and adequate management. As a general rule, if the fetus continues to maintain a stable baseline and a reassuring variability, the risk of hypoxia to the central organs is very unlikely. However, the general principles that should guide clinical management are outlined in the table.

FIGO guidelines clearly state that when fetal hypoxia/acidosis is anticipated or suspected (suspicious and pathological tracings) and action is required to avoid adverse neonatal outcome, this does not necessarily mean an immediate caesarean section or instrumental vaginal delivery. The underlying cause for the appearance of the pattern can frequently be identified and the situation reversed with subsequent recovery of adequate fetal oxygenation and return to a normal tracing.

Good clinical judgement is required to diagnose the underlying cause for a suspicious or pathological CTG to judge the reversibility of the conditions with which it is associated and to determine the timing of delivery with the objective of avoiding prolonged fetal hypoxia/ acidosis as well as unnecessary obstetric intervention. Additional methods may be used to evaluate fetal oxygenation. When a suspicious or worsening CTG pattern is identified, the underlying cause should be addressed before a pathological tracing develops. If the situation does not revert and the pattern continues to deteriorate, consideration needs to be given for further evaluation or rapid delivery if a pathological pattern ensues.

During the second stage of labour, due to the additional effect of maternal pushing, hypoxia/acidosis may develop more rapidly. Therefore, urgent action should be undertaken to relieve the situation, including discontinuation of maternal pushing, and if there is no improvement, delivery should be expedited

Implementation of FIGO Guidelines in Clinical Practice

It is important that midwives and obstetricians employ the principles of fetal physiology and physiological response to intrapartum hypoxic stress prior to taking action after classifying the CTG trace as normal, suspicious or pathological. Baseline FHR should be considered in accordance with the gestational age of the fetus (i.e. a postterm fetus would be expected to have a lower baseline heart rate), as well as a rise in baseline heart rate due to catecholamine surge may need action, even though the upper limit of the threshold (i.e. 160 bpm) is not breached. It is important to determine the presence of cycling and types of hypoxia while interpreting CTG traces.

Even if the CTG is classified as pathological, in the presence of a stable baseline FHR and reassuring variability, usually no operative intervention is required other than careful observation and/or alleviation of the cause of hypoxic or mechanical stress. Conversely, a fetus with a 'normal CTG' may require an operative intervention (e.g. clinical chorioamnionitis with failure to progress in labour). The presence of meconium staining of amniotic fluid and ongoing clinical chorioamnionitis may result in neurological injury secondary to meconium aspiration syndrome and inflammatory brain damage, even if the CTG trace is not 'pathological'. The use of tocolytics may help improve utero-placental circulation if acute accidents such as placental abruption or uterine rupture are excluded.

Further Reading

1. Ayres-de-Campos D, Spong CY, Chandraharan E; FIGO Intrapartum Fetal Monitoring Expert Consensus Panel. FIGO consensus guidelines on intrapartum fetal monitoring: Cardiotocography. *Int J Gynaecol Obstet*. 2015;131(1):13–24. www.ijgo.org/article/S0020-7292%2815%2900395-1/fulltext

Answers to Exercises

Chapter 3. Physiology of Fetal Heart Rate Control and Types of Intrapartum Hypoxia

1. How would you classify the decelerations in Figures 3.7, 3.8 and 3.9? Why?

Answer

1. *Typical variable decelerations.* This is because they vary in size, shape and in relation to uterine contractions (i.e. variable) and are characterized by a sharp drop and sharp recovery to the baseline (<60 seconds) due to 'baroreceptor reflex response'. Also note the presence of shouldering.

   Late decelerations. Unlike variable decelerations, a drop in FHR is more gradual, and more importantly, the recovery to normal baseline occurs late, even after the contraction has subsided. This is because they are mediated through chemoreceptors, and fresh oxygenated blood needs to 'wash out' all the accumulated carbon dioxide and metabolic acids during uterine relaxation to remove the stimulus.

   Atypical (or complicated) variable decelerations. Note the sharp drop and rapid recovery (i.e. variable mediated through the baroreceptor reflex), but the duration of these decelerations last for >60 seconds. In addition, 'biphasic pattern' is also seen with total loss of shouldering.

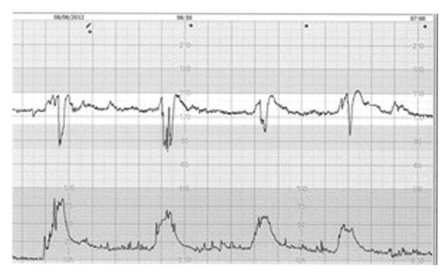

Figure 3.7

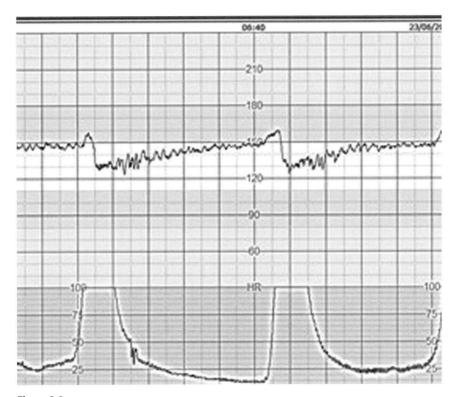

Figure 3.8

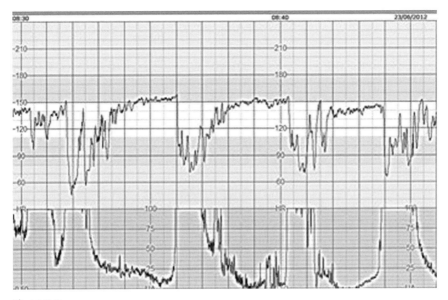

Figure 3.9

Chapter 5. Applying Fetal Physiology to Interpret CTG Traces: Predicting the NEXT Change

CTG Exercise A

1. A 32-year-old primigravida was admitted with spontaneous onset of labour at 39 weeks plus 3 days of gestation. On vaginal examination, her cervix was 6 cm dilated with evidence of spontaneous rupture of membranes. Clear amniotic fluid was draining and the presenting part was at the level of ischial spines. FHR was 128 bpm on intermittent auscultation. Four hours later, she was still found to be 6 cm dilated and, therefore, oxytocin infusion was commenced.

     Time to predict the NEXT change on the CTG trace:

   a. What changes would you expect to see on the CTG trace after commencement of oxytocin infusion if the fetus is exposed to an evolving hypoxic stress?
   b. If hypoxia worsens, what would you expect to see happening to the decelerations?
   c. If oxytocin infusion is further increased and hypoxia worsens, what would be expected to be seen on the CTG trace?
   d. What would you expect to see on the CTG trace?
   e. After the onset of cerebral decompensation (loss of baseline FHR variability), if oxytocin infusion was further increased, what is the next (i.e. last) organ to fail and what would you observe on the CTG trace?

Answers

1. a. Decelerations will be noted as the first sign of hypoxic stress as the fetus attempts to protect its myocardium by reducing myocardial workload. If the hypoxic stress continues, accelerations will disappear to conserve oxygen and nutrients by reducing nonessential body movements (somatic nervous system activity). A further increase in hypoxic stress secondary to oxytocin infusion may result in fetal catecholamine surge to increase the baseline FHR to perfuse vital organs at a faster rate and also to obtain more oxygen from the placenta (Figure 5.6).

   b. Decelerations would become wider and deeper (Figure 5.7) as the fetus attempts to protect its myocardium for prolonged periods of time to maintain a positive energy balance. This is similar to a progressive increase in the rate and depth of respiration in adults with prolonged and strenuous exercise to oxygenate the heart.

   As long as the baseline FHR and variability are normal and the time spent on the baseline is more than the time spent during decelerations (Figure 5.7), the central organs are well perfused and the risk of fetal acidosis is very low.

   c. The fetal reserve of a well-grown, term fetus with normal adrenal glands may release more catecholamines to compensate and, therefore, may further increase its heart rate (Figure 5.8), whereas a fetus with limited reserves (e.g. intrauterine growth restriction) may rapidly decompensate, leading to a loss of baseline FHR variability. Unfortunately, clinicians had failed to notice the increase in baseline FHR secondary to catecholamine surge and, therefore, wrongly classified the CTG trace as 'normal'. They had considered ongoing decelerations as 'typical' variable decelerations and,

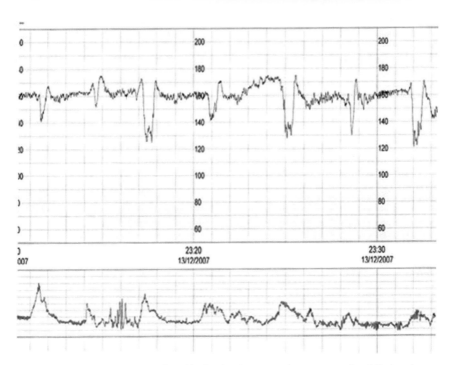

Figure 5.6 Note the appearance of variable decelerations secondary to repeated umbilical cord compression, loss of accelerations and an increase in baseline FHR secondary to catecholamine surge, 4 hours after commencing oxytocin infusion. Note that the baseline FHR is stable and the variability is reassuring, which indicates good oxygenation of the central organs.

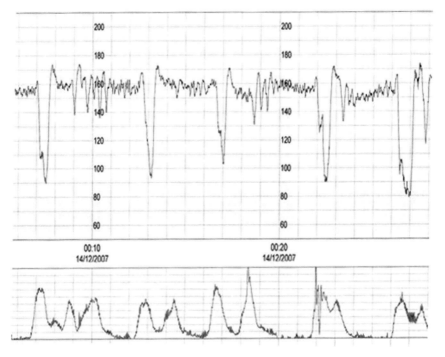

Figure 5.7 Note that within 40 minutes of continuation of hypoxic stress, decelerations have become wider and deeper. The baseline FHR is stable and the baseline variability is reassuring, indicating adequate oxygenation of the central organs.

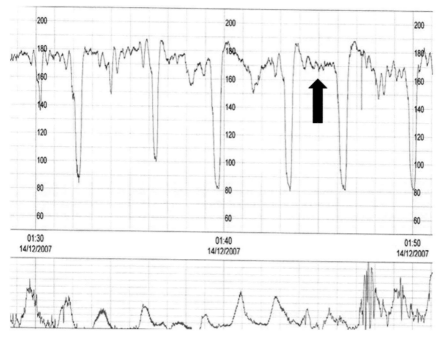

Figure 5.8 Note a further increase in FHR to above 170 bpm, which is significantly higher than the baseline FHR on admission (128 bpm), which indicates the degree of catecholamine surge. The fetus is still attempting to maintain a stable baseline FHR and a reassuring variability (arrow), but rapid decompensation may ensue if oxytocin infusion is further increased.

therefore, opined that the CTG would become 'suspicious' only if these decelerations persisted for >90 minutes, according to NICE guidelines. Therefore, they further increased the rate of oxytocin infusion.

d. Depending on the fetal reserve, either a further increase in FHR due to the release of catecholamines or a reduction of baseline FHR variability secondary to the onset of fetal decompensation.

The CTG trace clearly shows a final attempt by the fetus to maintain oxygenation by increasing the baseline heart rate to 200 bpm (Figure 5.9). However, such marked tachycardia would result in reduced ventricular filling time leading to reduced cardiac output and resultant reduction in carotid blood supply. The onset of cerebral hypoxia and acidosis will result in a reduction in baseline FHR variability (Figure 5.9).

The onset of reduction in baseline variability requires urgent action to improve utero-placental circulation. These include immediate stopping of oxytocin infusion, rapid infusion of intravenous fluids to dilute oxytocin concentration in maternal circulation and changes in position to relieve umbilical cord compression and use of tocolytics, if variability does not improve with initial measures. Unfortunately, due to a total lack of understanding of fetal physiological response to an evolving hypoxic stress, clinicians continued to increase oxytocin infusion to achieve 'progress' of labour and also commenced maternal active pushing to expedite delivery.

e. The last organ to fail is the myocardium (i.e. the heart) as persistent baseline fetal tachycardia increases the workload of the heart and reduces its own blood supply

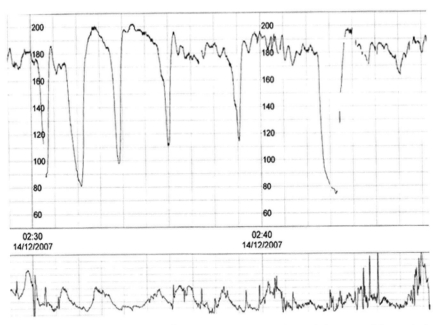

Figure 5.9 Note the final attempt by a fetus to maintain oxygenation to vital organs and the onset of reduction in baseline variability suggesting that this attempt was unsuccessful and that the fetus had moved from compensation to decompensation.

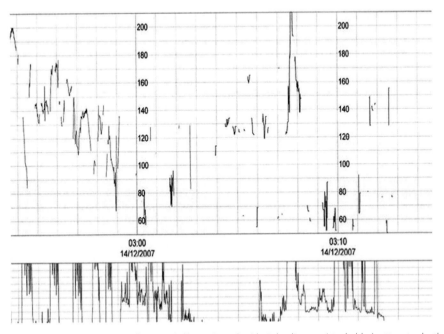

Figure 5.10 Note the onset of myocardial hypoxia and acidosis leading to a 'stepladder' pattern to death.

due to a reduction in cardiac relaxation time. In addition, increasing the rate of oxytocin infusion during the second stage of labour and maternal active pushing can result in a rapidly evolving hypoxia leading to fetal decompensation. The onset of myocardial hypoxia and acidosis will be characterized by the 'stepladder' pattern to death (Figure 5.10), culminating in terminal bradycardia.

CTG Exercise B

1. A primigravida was admitted with spontaneous onset of labour at 40 weeks plus 6 days of gestation. Oxytocin was commenced for failure to progress at 5 cm dilatation, 2 hours after artificial rupture of membranes. Clear amniotic fluid was noted and CTG trace was commenced. Apply '8Cs' on the CTG trace (Figure 5.11).

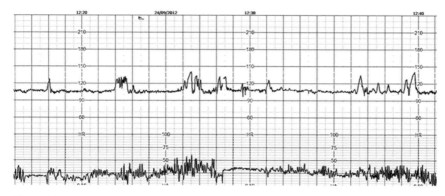

Figure 5.11

2. What features would you expect to see on the CTG trace if this fetus is exposed to a gradually evolving hypoxic stress?
3. After protecting the myocardium, how will the fetus redistribute oxygen to central organs? What would you expect to see on the CTG trace?
4. What would happen to ongoing decelerations as hypoxia progresses?
5. What would you expect to see if there is onset of fetal decompensation?

Answers

1. **Clinical picture** – Primigravida on oxytocin for augmentation of labour

   Cumulative uterine activity – Difficult to determine. However, there are no ongoing decelerations suggestive of hypoxia

   Cycling – Present

   Central nervous system oxygenation – Stable baseline FHR and a reassuring variability suggestive of good oxygenation of fetal myocardium and autonomic nerve centres in the brain

   Catecholamine surge – None

   Chemo- or baroreceptor decelerations – None

   Cascade – Continue monitoring

Consider the NEXT change on the CTG trace – Onset of decelerations

2. Onset of decelerations (Figure 5.12) to protect fetal myocardium so as to maintain a positive energy balance.
   Figure 5.12: Note the appearance of decelerations.

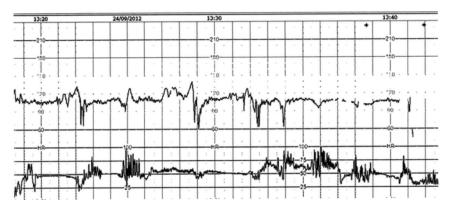

Figure 5.12

3. The fetus will release catecholamines to redistribute blood from nonessential to essential organs as well as compensatory tachycardia to supply vital organs and to get oxygenated blood from the placenta at a faster rate. Note a gradually increasing baseline from 110 to 130 bpm secondary to catecholamine surge with ongoing decelerations (Figure 5.13), which could be easily missed.
   As national guidelines give a wide range (110–160 bpm), such an increase in baseline FHR may be easily missed, if one does not understand fetal physiological response to hypoxic stress.

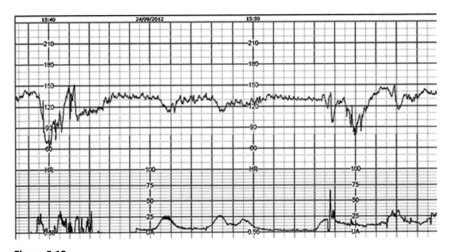

Figure 5.13

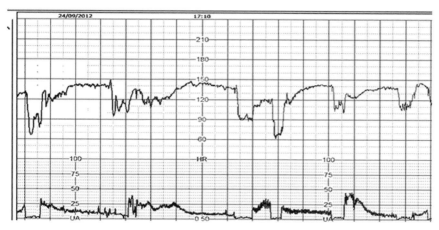

Figure 5.14

4. The decelerations would become wider and deeper (Figure 5.14) with a further increase in baseline FHR due to catecholamine release to help oxygenate the vital organs.

   Figure 5.14: Note the decelerations becoming wider and deeper with progressively worsening hypoxic stress and an attempt by the fetus to compensate for this by further increasing the baseline fetal FHR secondary to catecholamine surge.

   However, the end of the CTG trace shows loss of baseline FHR variability illustrating the onset of decompensation. Rapid action is required to improve fetal oxygenation (i.e. stopping oxytocin and rapid infusion of intravenous fluids, changing maternal position and use of tocolytics, if variability does not improve with initial measures).

5. Loss of baseline FHR variability due to lack of oxygen to the brain (Figure 5.14). If no action is taken, myocardial hypoxia and acidosis will ensue leading to a stepwise pattern to death culminating in terminal bradycardia.

Chapter 8. Intermittent (Intelligent) Auscultation in the Low-Risk Setting

1. A 30-year-old primigravida presented with spontaneous labour at 39 weeks, having had a low-risk pregnancy. On vaginal examination, cervix was 6 cm dilated, fully effaced with the presenting part 2 to the ischial spines. Bulging membranes were felt. She is requesting entonox for analgesia.
   a. Is CTG monitoring indicated? Why?
   b. On auscultation of the fetal heart, for 1 minute after the contraction, the heart rate is heard at an average of 140 bpm. Using the principles of IA, what is your diagnosis? What other information do you need?
   c. What is your action plan following assessment?
   d. Before the next vaginal examination was due, decelerations were heard using a hand-held Doppler following a contraction. What would your actions be?

2. Having had a low-risk pregnancy, with normal scans, a 25-year-old primigravida presented with spontaneous labour at 41 weeks and 2 days. Spontaneous rupture of membranes was confirmed on speculum 14 hours ago. On vaginal examination, cervix was found to be 5 cm dilated, fully effaced, and well applied to the fetal head, with the presenting part 2 to the ischial spines. Clear liquor is noted.
   a. On auscultation of FHR for 1 minute after a contraction, the fetal heart is heard at a rate of 150 bpm. What other information do you need?
   b. What are the possible causes of the findings?
   c. Is CTG monitoring indicated? Why?

Answers

1. a. No. The woman is 'low risk', and therefore the use of CTG in this situation will not improve the neonatal outcome, but may increase the likelihood of unnecessary interventions.
   b. Normal baseline rate, but need to listen for an acceleration to exclude chronic hypoxia. Have the fetal movements been normal? The care provider should listen following a contraction to ensure that there are no (late) decelerations.
   c. If the aforementioned initial assessment is normal, plan for intermittent auscultation every 15 minutes in first stage, every 5 minutes in second stage. Mobilize, analgesia as required, reassess progress in 4 hours. If no accelerations are heard, fetal movements are reported as reduced, or decelerations are heard during intermittent auscultation, then a CTG is indicated.
   d. Assess vaginally to exclude imminent delivery and commence CTG. If normal for 20 minutes, then discontinue and return to intermittent auscultation.

2. a. Are fetal movements normal? Has acceleration been heard? Are there any decelerations? Have there been any previous CTGs or antenatal recording of the fetal heart for comparison, as 150 bpm is high for this gestation although within normal limits by national guidelines. What are the maternal observations? Is there any offensive liquor?
   b. Chorioamnionitis; maternal tachycardia (secondary to pyrexia or dehydration); evolving hypoxia; normal rate for the individual fetus.
   c. Yes, as this is a high baseline rate for this gestation (although within national guidelines), and there is already a risk factor for sepsis (prolonged rupture of membrane [PROM] 14 hours). If all observations are satisfactory and evidence shows that this may be a normal rate (e.g. previous CTG with baseline at 150 bpm), then consider discontinuing. Continuous monitoring is indicated if PROM >24 hours, maternal temperature, suspected chorioamnionitis.

Chapter 10. Role of Uterine Contractions and Intrapartum Reoxygenation Ratio

1. A 25-year-old primigravida at 39 weeks of gestation presented with a history of spontaneous onset of labour. On vaginal examination, her cervix was 6 cm dilated with the presence of grade 2 meconium staining of the amniotic fluid.

Four hours later, her labour was augmented with syntocinon (oxytocin) infusion as there was no progress of labour, and ongoing uterine contractions were deemed inadequate.

Two hours after commencement of syntocinon infusion, uterine contractions were occurring 6 in 10 minutes each lasting 60 seconds on the CTG trace (Figure 10.2).

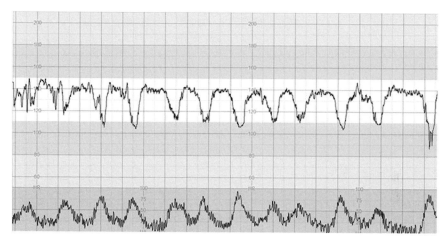

Figure 10.2

a. What is your differential diagnosis?
b. Is CTG monitoring indicated?
c. What abnormalities will be noted on the CTG based on the differential diagnosis?
d. What is your management?
e. What will be noticed on the CTG trace if treatment is instituted?

Answers

1. a. Uterine hyperstimulation
   b. Yes, it is important to monitor the FHR continuously if oxytocin infusion is used and/or in the presence of meconium.
   c. Frequent uterine contractions, less relaxation time in between contractions with a stable baseline rate of 140 and a reassuring baseline variability. Repeated variable decelerations with a stable baseline FHR and reassuring variability suggestive of compensated fetal stress response.
   d. Reduce oxytocin infusion in the first instance and observe for reduction in the depth and duration of variable decelerations and increased relaxation time. If no such changes are observed within 3–5 minutes (half-life of oxytocin), then oxytocin infusion should be stopped. Intravenous fluids may be administered to dilute oxytocin and to improve placental circulation. Terbutaline should be administered if no improvement is noted with initial measures.
   e. Disappearance of decelerations, more time on baseline and reappearance of accelerations (Figure 10.3)
      Figure 10.3: CTG trace 40 minutes after stopping oxytocin infusion. Note the disappearance of decelerations and appearance of accelerations.

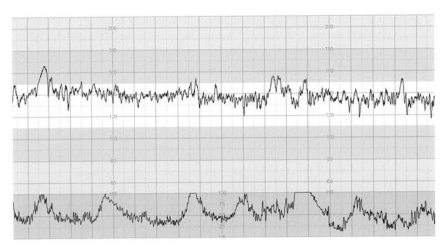

Figure 10.3

Chapter 11. Intrapartum Monitoring of a Preterm Fetus

1. A 24-year-old primigravida presents at 28 weeks with reduced fetal movements. The CTG trace is shown in the figure.
    a. Classify the CTG applying the '8Cs' approach.
    b. What are the specific features different from those of a term fetus?
    c. What changes would you expect to see if you repeat the CTG in 4 weeks' time?
    d. How would you assess fetal well-being at this stage of pregnancy?

Answers

1. a. **Clinical picture:** Preterm fetus, 28 weeks. Reduced fetal movements.
        Cumulative uterine activity: Not registered in this case.
        Cycling of FHR: This is a preterm fetus and FHR cycling may not be evident. The autonomic nervous system is not fully developed at this stage, and therefore, an apparent reduction variability may be seen due to unopposed activity of the sympathetic nervous system without opposing effect of the parasympathetic nervous system.
        Central organ oxygenation: It is difficult to assess in preterm fetuses as this is shown by the variability which, as mentioned earlier, is expected to be reduced in preterm fetuses due to immaturity.
        Catecholamine surge: The predominant component of the autonomic nervous system is the sympathetic component, and therefore, an increased baseline rate (150–160 bpm) would be expected.
        Chemo- or baroreceptor decelerations: There are some baroreceptor decelerations which in preterm fetuses can be due to fetal movements.
        Cascade: This patient has presented with reduced fetal movements. An ultrasound scan to assess fetal growth and Doppler and computerized CTG are more appropriate to assess fetal well-being.

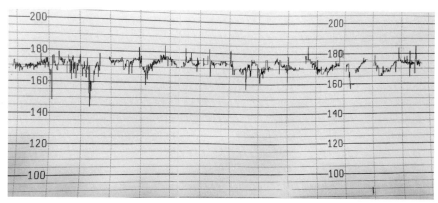

Figure 11.1

b. Baseline heart rate is increased (150–160 bpm) due to the predominant effect of the sympathetic nervous system without opposing effect of the parasympathetic nervous system. Due to immaturity of the somatic nervous system, accelerations may be absent or may have a low amplitude without any clinical significance.

The variability can be reduced due to immaturity of the autonomic nervous system. The presence of variable or early decelerations is indeterminate usually secondary to compression of the umbilical cord during fetal movements due to the absence of the Wharton jelly and should not trigger delivery on a preterm fetus.

c. Consider the NEXT Change on the CTG if pregnancy is allowed to continue The baseline rate will decrease to ranges between 140 and 150 bpm, as the parasympathetic system develops. For the same reason, variability will also increase as the gestation advances. Accelerations would become more pronounced with the maturation of the somatic nervous system.

d. In preterm fetuses, fetal well-being is more reliably assessed by Doppler and short-term variability on computerized CTG as the usual features (baseline FHR, variability and decelerations) analysed are unreliable in fetuses <32 weeks.

Chapter 12. Role of Chorioamnionitis and Infection

1. A primigravida was admitted for induction of labour at 41 weeks + 3 days of gestation. She had no antenatal risk factors. CTG trace was commenced (Figure 12.3).

   a. How would you classify the CTG trace?
   b. What is your management plan?

   A plan was made for expectant management and the maternal pulse rate was noted to be 108 bpm.

   c. What is the likely diagnosis?
   d. What is your management plan?
   e. What are the signs and symptoms you would be anticipating in this case?

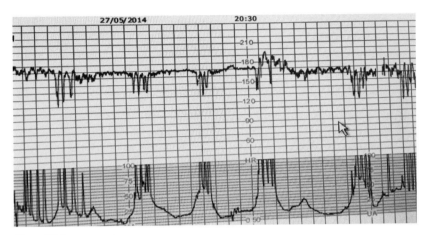

Figure 12.3

A plan was made to continue with labour. Three hours later, maternal temperature was recorded as 38.2°C. Paracetamol and intravenous antibiotics were administered. Six hours later, cervix was found to be 4 cm dilated and artificial rupture of membranes was carried out and meconium staining of amniotic fluid was noted.

   f. What is your diagnosis?

   g. What is your management plan and why?

Answers

1. a. According to guidelines, this would be a suspicious CTG as the baseline FHR is between 160 and 180 bpm. The absence of cycling (alternative periods of activity and quiescence) has been persisting for >40 minutes.

    b. The baseline FHR would be expected to be closer to the lower limit of normal (i.e. 110 bpm) at 41 weeks + 3 days due to parasympathetic dominance. Although the absence of accelerations during established labour is of uncertain significance, accelerations should always be observed during the antenatal period or in early labour. In addition, the absence of cycling reflects depression of the central nervous system centres (sympathetic and parasympathetic that control the heart rate). Therefore, in view of an increased baseline FHR and absence of cycling, a strong index of clinical suspicion of subclinical chorioamnionitis should be made. In the absence of decelerations, chronic hypoxia is unlikely and maternal dehydration may cause fetal tachycardia but not absence of cycling or loss of accelerations.

      Therefore, a careful observation of other features of chorioamnionitis (maternal tachycardia, maternal pyrexia, meconium staining of amniotic fluid) should be carried out. One needs to remember that hypoxia secondary to the onset of uterine contractions worsens neurological injury in the presence of fetal infection.

    c. Onset of maternal tachycardia strongly suggests ongoing subclinical chorioamnionitis.

d. If the CTG trace continues to show increased baseline FHR as compared to expected 110 bpm and loss of accelerations and cycling, delivery should be recommended. This is because the patient is a primigravida and delivery is not imminent and continuation of labour would not only result in prolonged exposure of the fetal brain to inflammatory mediators, but it may also result in additional hypoxic stress secondary to uterine contractions.

Note uterine irritability and presence of episodes of 'saltatory pattern' on the CTG trace suggestive of possible chorioamnionitis. Saltatory pattern has been described in cases of fetal infection (autonomic instability due to increased temperature).

e. Maternal tachycardia, meconium staining of amniotic fluid and offensive vaginal discharge.

f. Clinical chorioamnionitis – beyond any reasonable doubt.

g. As delivery is not imminent and she is a primigravida, an emergency 'category 2' caesarean section (aim to deliver within the next 60 minutes) should be performed. This is because continuation of labour may lead to neurological damage and decompensation of the brain. Inflammatory damage to the myocardium may result in myocardial dysfunction and cardiac membrane damage leading to terminal bradycardia.

The absence of variability and of cycling are hallmarks of decompensation of the central nervous system secondary hypoxia, acidosis and inflammatory brain damage, and continuation of labour when delivery is not imminent may lead to myocardial decompensation and terminal bradycardia.

Comment: This case illustrates the role of CTG in highlighting ongoing subclinical chorioamnionitis and the importance of avoiding additional hypoxic stress (prostaglandins, artificial rupture of membranes and use of oxytocin to augment labour) unless fetal well-being could be absolutely determined based on the features observed on the CTG trace. An increase in baseline FHR (albeit within the normal range of 110–160 bpm) for the given gestation with absence of accelerations and cycling are ominous features, and delivery should always be considered if it is not imminent. Continuation of labour may result in additive detrimental effects of hypoxic stress (uterine contractions and umbilical cord compression) on a fetus already experiencing inflammatory damage and thereby may potentiate neurological injury.

Chapter 14. Intrapartum Bleeding

1. A 36-year-old primigravida presented with a history of painless vaginal bleeding with reduced fetal movements at 40 weeks of gestation. On examination, the abdomen was soft and nontender and FHR was 160 bpm. On speculum examination, fresh vaginal bleeding was noted.

   a. What is your differential diagnosis?
   b. Is CTG monitoring indicated?
   c. What abnormalities on the CTG would be expected based on your differential diagnosis?

d. CTG was commenced and the following features were noted (Figure 14.5). What is your diagnosis?
e. What is your management?

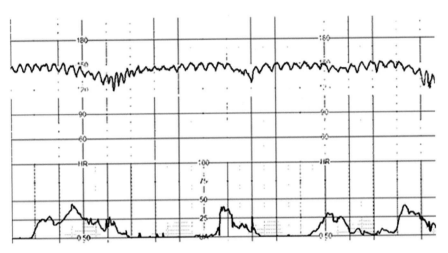

Figure 14.5

Answers

1. a. Revealed abruption, unrecognized placenta praevia, local causes and vasa praevia.
   b. Yes, it is important to exclude fetal hypoxia if bleeding was of fetal origin.
   c. Abruption – recurrent late decelerations with loss of baseline FHR variability. Vasa praevia – atypical sinusoidal pattern ('poole shark teeth pattern').
   d. Atypical sinusoidal pattern (poole shark teeth pattern) and therefore fetomaternal haemorrhage.

      Apply 8Cs while interpreting CTG traces:

      Clinical picture – unexplained vaginal bleeding and reduced fetal movements

      Cumulative uterine activity (frequency and duration) – 5 in 10 minutes

      Cycling of FHR – none

      Central organ oxygenation – baseline is stable but loss of variability with atypical sinusoidal pattern, also called the 'poole shark teeth pattern'

      Catecholamine surge – yes, baseline is higher than expected at 40 weeks

      Chemo- or baroreceptor decelerations – none

      Cascade – High risk with evidence of CNS hypoxia likely from fetomaternal haemorrhage – needs immediate delivery

      Consider next change – myocardial decompensation and terminal bradycardia
   e. Clear explanation to the woman regarding the possibility of ongoing fetal hypoxia and hypotension secondary to fetal bleeding. Immediate delivery (category 1 C-section) and inform the neonatal team regarding the need to check haemoglobin and for immediate fluid resuscitation and blood transfusion in view of likely fetal hypotension.

This patient had an emergency caesarean section and a ruptured vasa praevia (Figure 14.4).

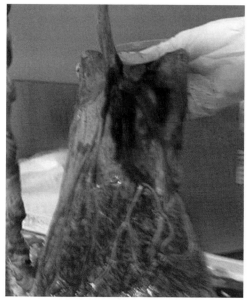

Figure 14.4 Note the ruptured vasa praevia in a case with an atypical sinusoidal pattern with a 'jagged edge' resembling 'Poole Shark Teeth'.

Chapter 15. Labour with a Uterine Scar: The Role of CTG

1. A 36-year-old gravida 2 para 1 with a previous caesarean section for failure to progress in labour was admitted with spontaneous onset of labour. Cervix was 6 cm dilated and the presenting part was at 0 station and the CTG trace was classified as normal. Oxytocin was commenced at 23:00 hours for failure to progress in labour as her cervix had remained 6 cm 2 hours after artificial rupture of membranes.

    a. Classify the CTG trace (using the '8C' format).
    b. What are effects of oxytocin on myometrial contractions and what changes would you observe on the CTG trace?
    c. Consider the CTG trace from 02:58 hours.
        1. What is the type of hypoxia?
        2. What are the differential diagnoses?
        3. What immediate actions would you take?
    d. What is the likelihood of the observed CTG change to return back to normal in this case?
    e. What would you expect to see in the umbilical cord gases if delivery was accomplished within 20 minutes of the onset of this acute, prolonged decelerations?

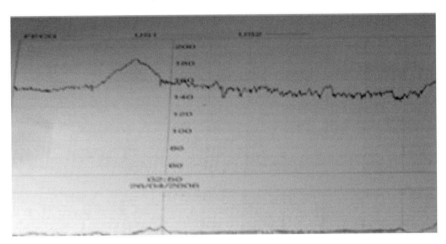

Figure 15.1

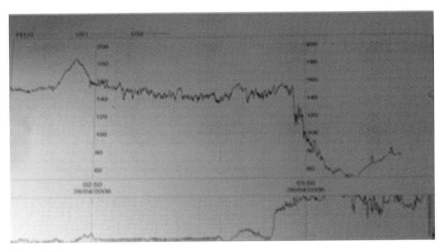

Figure 15.2

Answers

1. a. Apply 8Cs while interpreting CTG traces.

   Clinical picture – previous caesarean section, oxytocin augmentation

   Cumulative uterine activity (frequency and duration) – no contractions recorded at present

   Cycling of FHR – present; presence of periods of accelerations and good variability alternating with periods of quiescence with reduced variability

   Central organ oxygenation – good variability reflecting good oxygenation of the central nervous system (brain)

Catecholamine surge – no, baseline is about 145 bpm

Chemo- or baroreceptor decelerations – no decelerations present

Cascade – risk of uterine rupture in the presence of a uterine scar and oxytocin augmentation

Consider next change – In the presence of oxytocin augmentation, if there is a uterine dehiscence, repetitive decelerations will be recorded; however, if there is a complete uterine, a prolonged deceleration with loss of variability within the first 3 minutes will appear.

b. Oxytocin produces stronger and more frequent contractions. If oxytocin continues to be increased, uterine tachysystole/hypertonia on the 'toco' component may be observed and presence of decelerations on the 'cardiograph'.

If there is uterine dehiscence, repetitive decelerations and loss of variability will appear; and if it is a complete rupture, a prolonged deceleration would be observed.

c. 1. Acute hypoxia
    2. Differential diagnosis includes:
       • Uterine scar rupture
       • Cord prolapse
       • Abruption
       • Iatrogenic causes (oxytocin causing hypertonia, epidural causing hypotension)
    3. Stop oxytocin, prepare for an immediate delivery as there is loss of baseline variability within the first 3 minutes of deceleration and the clinical diagnosis is uterine rupture. In this case, the '3, 6, 9, 12, 15' rule cannot be applied. Immediate delivery is the appropriate management in this clinical scenario.

d. In the presence of one of the three major accidents, prolonged deceleration would not be expected to recover as fetal hypoxia can only get worse over time. If a prolonged deceleration is due to iatrogenic causes and in the absence of three major accidents, 90 percent of these decelerations will recover in 6 minutes within the onset of deceleration and 95 percent by 9 minutes.

e. The rate of fall in pH during acute hypoxia is 0.01 per minute. The CTG prior to the onset of prolonged deceleration was normal, and we would expect a normal pH of around 7.25. If the delivery is accomplished within 20 minutes, the pH will drop by 0.2 unit ($0.01 \times 20 = 0.2$), and therefore the umbilical cord arterial pH at birth would be expected to be around 7.05.

Chapter 16. Impact of Maternal Environment on Fetal Heart Rate

1. A 31-year-old primigravida presents to the labour ward at 37 weeks of gestation with a history of regular contractions. She was diagnosed with type 1 diabetes at the age of 11 and uses insulin pump therapy. Her HBA1c at booking was 56 mmol/mol and control has been difficult during pregnancy. She appears dehydrated and urine dipstick shows >3 ketones. On admission she is found to be 3 cm dilated and CTG monitoring is commenced. The following trace is observed:
    a. How would you classify the CTG?

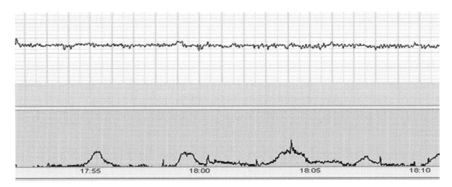

Figure 16.1

  b. What do you need to consider given her history and how might it impact upon the CTG?

  c. How will you manage her?

Answers

1. a. The CTG can be described using the 8Cs technique:

    Clinical picture: The mother is a poorly controlled type 1 diabetic in early labour. She is showing signs of diabetic ketoacidosis, a form of metabolic acidosis.

    Cumulative uterine activity: Contraction frequency is 2 in 10, and each contraction is lasting approximately 60 seconds in duration.

    Cycling: There is no evidence of cycling on this portion of the CTG.

    Central organ oxygenation: Baseline variability is reduced (between 3 and 5), indicating that central nervous system centres (sympathetic and parasympathetic) are depressed. Causes include fetal sleep, drugs (opiates), hypoxia and acidosis.

    Chemoreceptor/baroreceptor decelerations: There is no evidence of decelerations mediated by either chemo- or baroreceptors. However, in cases of severe maternal acidosis, loss of variability may occur before the onset of decelerations.

    Catecholamine surge: The baseline heart rate is stable, without the rise that usually appears in cases of gradually evolving hypoxia. However, in cases of severe maternal acidosis, reduced baseline variability may be the first change seen on the CTG trace, even in the absence of acidosis.

    Compute and cascade: There is evidence of severe maternal acidosis in the form of diabetic ketoacidosis, which may be causing the CTG changes. A full assessment of the mother is required, and treatment of ketoacidosis should be urgently instituted to optimize maternal condition

    Consider next change: Given that central nervous system centres are already depressed secondary to passive transfer of maternal acidosis, any further hypoxic stress will cause myocardial decompensation and prolonged deceleration.

  b. There is evidence of severe maternal acidosis; in such fetuses, baseline variability may be lost before the onset of decelerations and a rise in baseline FHR.

  c. Management involves treatment of the cause of CTG change. A full assessment of the mother must be made by performing blood glucose and blood gas testing. Urea and electrolytes should also be checked and IV (intravenous) access obtained. If diabetic ketoacidosis is confirmed, the mother should be treated using an insulin/dextrose infusion, with careful monitoring of potassium levels. Care should be multidisciplinary, with involvement from anaesthetic and medical teams.

Chapter 17. Use of CTG with Induction and Augmentation of Labour

1. A 30-year-old, G2 P1, previous caesarean section is being induced for postdates (41 + 4 weeks of gestation). She had prostaglandin pessary inserted for 24 hours, following which she had an artificial rupture of membranes (ARMs) that showed meconium grade 1. Two hours later, she was started on oxytocin infusion. Oxytocin has been augmented every 30 minutes as per protocol. CTG trace before the ARM was normal with a baseline FHR of 130 bpm, variability of 10–15 bpm, presence of accelerations with no decelerations and she had two contractions in 10 minutes.

   CTG after 8 hours of oxytocin augmentation shows the following features.

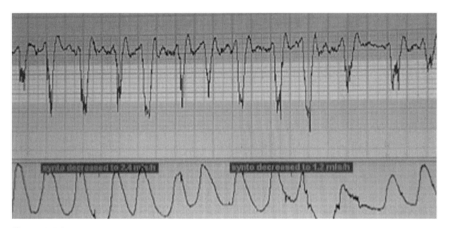

Figure 17.2

   a. What is your diagnosis?
   b. What is your management?
   c. What other complications do you expect?

Answers

1. a. Apply 8Cs while interpreting CTG traces:

   Clinical picture: induction of labour followed by oxytocin augmentation; previous caesarean section; meconium grade 1; postterm fetus

   Cumulative uterine activity (frequency and duration): 6 in 10 minutes

   Cycling of FHR: none

   Central organ oxygenation: good variability in between decelerations reflecting good oxygenation of the central nervous system (brain)

Catecholamine surge – yes, baseline is higher than expected (160 bpm) at 41 + 4 weeks and was previously recorded.

Chemo- or baroreceptor decelerations – baroreceptor deceleration due to umbilical cord compression; note the shouldering before and after deceleration, sharp fall of the FHR followed by a quick recovery to the normal baseline.

Cascade – risk of uterine rupture, meconium aspiration and fetal hypoxia if oxytocin augmentation continues

Consider next change – decelerations will become longer-lasting with delayed recovery, and there may be loss of shouldering. Onset of metabolic acidosis would result in delayed recovery to the baseline due to chemoreceptor-mediated response.

b. Stop/reduce oxytocin infusion. Consider tocolysis if frequency of contractions persists and there is no improvement on the CTG trace.

c. Uterine rupture as patient has a previous caesarean section. Meconium aspiration syndrome and if above interventions are delayed and if fetal decompensation ensues, fetal hypoxic-ischaemic encephalopathy (HIE).

Chapter 19. Unusual Fetal Heart Rate Patterns: Sinusoidal and Saltatory Patterns

1. A 35-year-old primigravida presents at 38 weeks of gestation with abdominal pain for 3 hours and reduced fetal movements with no vaginal bleeding. On examination, uterine contractions were palpated and the cervix was fully effaced, 2 cm dilated.

a. What is your differential diagnosis?

b. Is a CTG indicated?

c. She was re-examined in 4 hours and established to be in labour. She was later commenced on oxytocin for confirmed delay in the first stage of labour. Vaginal examination after 4 hours of oxytocin demonstrated that she was 8 cm dilated. Describe the CTG at this stage (Figure 19.3). Do you have any concerns?

d. She opted for an epidural anesthesia and is now fully dilated and has had a 2-hour passive descent. A repeat vaginal examination suggests that she is fully dilated with the fetal head in occipito-anterior position, at station +1. A decision has been made

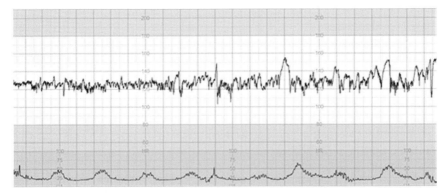

Figure 19.3

to start active pushing. She has been actively pushing for 20 minutes and CTG is given below (Figure 19.4). How would you describe the CTG?

e. What is your management plan based on the features observed on the CTG (Figure 19.4)?

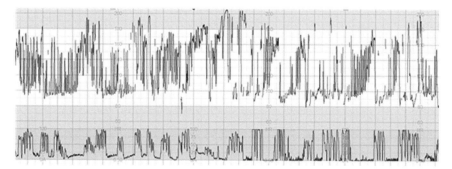

Figure 19.4

Answers

1. a. Early labour or a concealed placental abruption
   b. Yes – to exclude fetal hypoxia due to the history of reduced fetal movements
   c. No – baseline 130 bpm, variability 5–10 bpm, accelerations present, no decelerations. Overall normal CTG trace as autonomic and somatic nervous systems are well oxygenated with the presence of accelerations and cycling.
   d. Saltatory pattern – baseline FHR not defined, fetal heart baseline amplitude changes of >25 bpm with an oscillatory frequency of >6 per minute, occurring for 15 minutes
   e. Stop or reduce oxytocin to improve utero-placental circulation. In view of persisting saltatory pattern, the woman should be advised to stop active pushing in the second stage of labour to improve fetal oxygenation. CTG trace should be carefully observed for improvement (i.e. reappearance of a stable baseline FHR and reassuring variability). If no improvement is seen on the CTG trace, delivery should be accomplished. If immediate delivery is not possible, terbutaline should be administered while the woman is transferred to the operating theatre.

   Apply 8Cs while interpreting CTG traces:

   Clinical picture: 38 weeks presenting with abdominal pain and reduced fetal movements
   Cumulative uterine activity: 7 out of 10 minutes
   Cycling of FHR: absent
   Central organ oxygenation: absent stable baseline with variability >25 bpm
   Catecholamine surge: Yes, there are attempts to increase FHR to 180 bpm
   Chemo- or baroreceptor decelerations: Yes – repeated baroreceptor decelerations
   Cascade: Rapidly evolving hypoxia may lead to fetal overshoots and saltatory patterns; therefore, stop or reduce oxytocin or consider intravenous fluids or tocolysis.
   Consider next change: Myocardial decompensation and terminal bradycardia

Chapter 20. Intrauterine Resuscitation

1. A 29-year-old primigravida presented with spontaneous early labour at 39 + 4 weeks of gestation. She was commenced on oxytocin at 5 cm dilation for failure to progress. One hour later, her CTG trace (Figure 20.2) shows the following features.

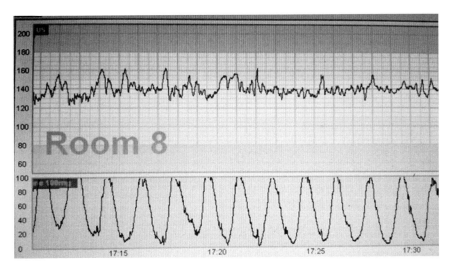

Figure 20.2

    a. What is your diagnosis?

       Two hours later, the CTG trace shows the following features (Figure 20.3):

    b. What is your diagnosis?
    c. What action will you take?

Answers

1. a. Uterine tachysystole – frequent/excessive uterine contractions with a normal cardiograph
   b. Uterine hyperstimulation – frequent/excessive uterine contractions with associated changes in the cardiograph (i.e. decelerations and/or changes in baseline)
   c. Stop oxytocin, consider fluid infusion to dilute oxytocin in systemic circulation, then reassess the CTG trace. If decelerations do not improve and a stable baseline FHR and variability are not maintained within 3–5 minutes (half-life of oxytocin), consider administration of tocolytics.

   Apply 8Cs to interpreting CTG traces:

   Clinical picture: oxytocin administration for failure to progress
   Cumulative uterine activity: 15 in 20 minutes
   Cycling of FHR: none
   Central organ oxygenation: initially good variability and return to baseline heart rate indicating good fetal reserve; however, with repeated stress, the baseline heart

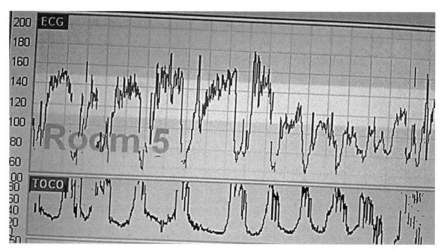

Figure 20.3

rate falls, suggestive of myocardial hypoxia and acidosis, and there is reduced variability within deceleration (hypoxia to the central nervous system)

Catecholamine surge: attempts at increasing the baseline heart rate, but due to repeated decelerations, a progressive reduction in baseline fetal heart rate is observed.

Chemo- or baroreceptor decelerations: baroreceptor decelerations with a sharp fall and a rapid recovery to the baseline. However, some decelerations demonstrate a delayed recovery suggestive of a co-existing chemoreceptor response as well. This is because, in addition to umbilical cord compression, oxytocin-induced sustained uterine contractions may also reduce utero-placental circulation leading to acidosis within the placental venous sinuses.

Cascade: suspected fetal compromise due to excessive uterine contractions

Consider next change: If no action is taken, due to progressive myocardial hypoxia and acidosis, prolonged deceleration culminating in a terminal bradycardia would ensue.

Management: Stop oxytocin, consider fluid infusion to dilute oxytocin in systemic circulation, and if CTG changes, do not normalize within 3–5 minutes (half-life of oxytocin), then consider administration of tocolytics.

Chapter 21. Management of Prolonged Decelerations and Bradycardia

1. A primigravida is induced at 41 + 5 weeks of gestation for postdates after a normal pregnancy. The CTG up to this point has been entirely normal with a baseline rate of 130 bpm and variability of 5–15 bpm. At 11:49, a deceleration begins and the attending midwife appropriately moves the mother into the left lateral position.
   You are called to the room at 11:54.
   a. What are the first steps you would take to assess the patient?
   b. What is the likely cause of this prolonged deceleration?

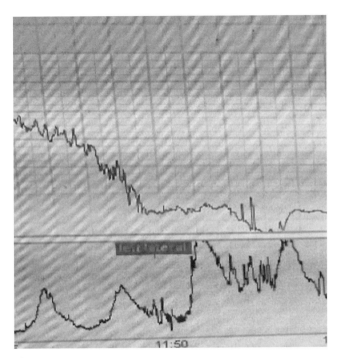

Figure 21.4

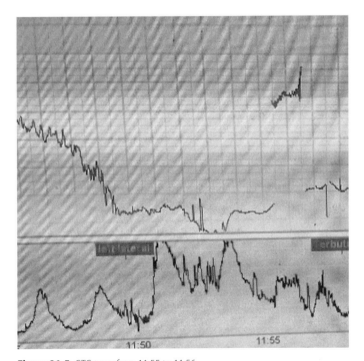

Figure 21.5 CTG trace from 11:55 to 11:56.

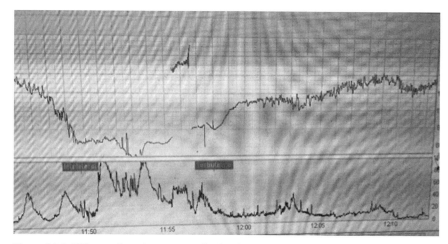

Figure 21.6 CTG trace after administration of terbutaline.

   c. What would your management be?

   d. What features on the CTG are reassuring?

   e. What features on the CTG are concerning?

      Now consider the trace again (Figure 21.5).

   f. What phenomenon is demonstrated at 11:55–11:56?

   g. Terbutaline is administered at 11:57. At 11:58 what would your next action be?

      Figure 21.6 shows the full trace indicating first recovery of the baseline and second restoration of normal variability suggesting an intact neurological system. The tocograph clearly demonstrates that the uterine activity has been temporarily abolished.

   h. What might you expect to see next on the CTG?

Answers

1. a. Examine the patient – BP and pulse, abdominal palpation and vaginal examination particularly for signs of abruption, cord prolapse or uterine rupture.

   b. Barring any evidence on physical examination of one of the three accidents, this deceleration is clearly in response to the prolonged uterine activity recorded on the tocograph and represents the fetal response to uterine hyperstimulation.

   c. Stop any syntocinon or consider removing prostaglandins if still present. Keep the patient in left lateral and correct any hypotension with intravenous fluids. Give terbutaline 250 mg subcutaneously as soon as possible.

   d. The preceding CTG was normal and the variability in the first 3 minutes is normal.

   e. The variability is lost as deceleration progresses and the FHR drops < 80.

   f. The FHR here is being doubled to give a falsely high reading. This would be clear to clinicians in the room if the 'sound' is turned on as a lower heart rate would be audible.

   g. At 1158, one should know that the fetus was normally oxygenated at the onset of deceleration and that the cause of deceleration is uterine tone, and therefore management of the underlying cause should be undertaken (i.e. uterine relaxation) while remaining prepared for an emergency delivery. It is expected that the baseline will recover within the next 1–2 minutes.

h. After deceleration, one would expect to see a rebound tachycardia; however, a strong fetus with good reserves will rapidly settle back down to the original baseline unless another source of stress causes need for further adrenaline release. Terbutaline itself may cause a transient fetal tachycardia.

Chapter 30. Medico-legal Issues with CTG

1. A 28-year-old gravida 2 is in spontaneous normal labour. She has no high-risk factors and she is in the active second stage of labour. She was monitored for audible abnormality of the FHR. Abdominally the fetus was estimated to be 3.8 kg and the head was 0/5th palpable. Vaginally there was clear amniotic fluid, she was fully dilated, and the occiput was in left occipito transverse position at station 0 to +1. There is ++ caput and ++ moulding. The CTG trace is shown in Figure 30.6.

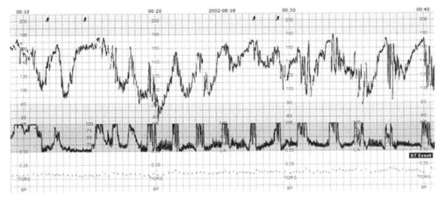

Figure 30.6

Describe your plan of action.
a. Observe for another hour
b. Perform FBS
c. Perform caesarean section
d. Perform instrumental delivery
e. Give acute tocolysis and await further descent

Answer

The decelerations are getting more and more prolonged (>2 minutes), and the FHR remains at the baseline rate only for about 30 seconds. The baseline variability has become salutatory suggestive of possible acute hypoxia. This would warrant immediate instrumental vaginal delivery in the next 15 to 30 minutes.

Index